Food Folklore
Tales and Truths
About What We Eat

D0469452

Written for
The American Dietetic Association
by Roberta Larson Duyff
MS, RD, CFCS

CHRONIMED PUBLISHING

Library of Congress Cataloging-in-Publication Data

Food folklore / The American Dietetic Association

    p.   cm.

Includes index.

ISBN 1-56561-168-3

Edited by: Jeff Braun
Cover Design: Terry Dugan Design
Text Design & Production: David Enyeart
Art/Production Manager: Claire Lewis

Printed in the United States of America

Published by
Chronimed Publishing
P.O. Box 59032
Minneapolis, MN 55459–0032

NOTICE: CONSULT A HEALTH CARE PROFESSIONAL Readers are advised to
seek the guidance of a licensed physician or health care professional
before making changes in health care regimens, since each individual case
or need may vary. This book is intended for informational purposes only
and is not for use as an alternative to appropriate medical care. While every
effort has been made to ensure that the information is the most current
available, new research findings, being released with increasing frequency,
may invalidate some data.

Food Folklore

Tales and Truths
About What We Eat

**Written for The American
Dietetic Association by**
Roberta Larson Duyff, MS, RD, CFCS
Duyff Associates
St. Louis, Missouri

**The American Dietetic Association
Reviewers:**

Barbara Allen, MS, RD
Carolee Bildsten, RD
National Center for Nutrition and
    Dietetics
Chicago, Illinois

Pamela Goyan Kittler, MS
Four Winds Food Specialists
Sunnyvale, California

Libby Mills, MS, RD
Diamond Crystal Specialty Foods, Inc.
Wilmington, Massachusetts

Kathryn P. Sucher, ScD, RD
San Jose State University
San Jose, California

Technical Editor:
Betsy Hornick, MS, RD
The American Dietetic Association
Chicago, Illinois

CHRONIMED PUBLISHING

THE AMERICAN DIETETIC ASSOCIATION is the largest group of food and health professionals in the world. As the advocate of the profession, the ADA serves the public by promoting optimal nutrition, health, and well-being.

For expert answers to your nutrition questions, call the ADA/ National Center for Nutrition and Dietetics Hot Line at (900) 225-5267. To listen to recorded messages or obtain a referral to a registered dietitian (RD) in your area, call (800) 366-1655. Visit the ADA's Website at www.eatright.org.

Contributors

We thank the following members of The American Dietetic Association for their contributions of common foodlore: Trudy Alexander, Barbara Anderson, Karen M. Baldacci, Erin DeSimone, Deanne Dolnick, Martha A. Erickson, Trudy Fedora, Jean Fischer, Lorri Fishman, Mary C. Friesz, Martha Grodrian, Shannon Helfert, Alice Henneman, Dorothy Humm, Barbara Ivens, Eliza Markidou, S. Mermelstein, Anne K. Milliken, Jennifer Nelson, Diane L. Olson, Kim Ouellette, Maureen Pestine, Jennifer Rauktis, Jaime Ruud, Jacalyn See, Lana Shepek, Cindy Silver, Lesley Stanford, Catherine Stein, E. Sturner, Cheryl Sullivan, Nancy Teigen, Lisa Theroux, Deanne Troyer, Barbara Truitt, Myra Waits, Madelyn L. Wheeler, Frances Wilkinson, Susan M. Williams, Allison Wolters.

Contents

Introduction 11

Aging and Longevity 15
Alcoholic Beverages 16
Anemia 16
Appetite 18
Arthritis 18
Body Weight 19
Bone Health 20
Breast-Feeding 21
Caffeine 22
Calories 23
Cancer 24
Carbohydrates 25
Child Feeding 26
Chocolate 27
Cholesterol in Food 28
Colds and Flu 28
Dairy Foods 30
Dehydration 31
Dental Health 31

Depression 32
Diabetes 32
Dietary Supplements 34
Digestion and Digestive Problems. 35
Eggs 37
Energy 37
Fast Food 38
Fasting 39
Fat. 39
Fertilizers and Pesticides 41
Fiber 41
Fingernails. 42
Fish and Seafood. 42
Fluids and Beverages. 43
Food Additives 43
Food Allergies and Sensitivities. 44
Food Cravings. 45
Food Labeling. 45
Food Preparation. 46
Food Safety and Foodborne Illness 47
Food Storage. 48
Fruit and Fruit Juice 49
Grain Products 50
Hair 51
Headaches 51
Health Foods. 52
Healthful Eating 52
Heart Health. 54
Herbs and Herbal Remedies 55
High Blood Pressure 56
Hyperactivity 57

Hypoglycemia 57
Infant Feeding 57
Irradiation 59
Legumes 59
Meal Skipping 60
Meat 60
Memory 61
Microwave Cooking 61
Minerals 61
Muscles and Strength 62
Nutrition Advice 63
Nuts and Seeds 63
Organic Foods 64
Physical Activity 64
Phytochemicals 65
Poultry 65
Pregnancy 65
Processed Foods 67
Productivity 67
Protein 67
Salt and Sodium 68
Sex and Fertility 69
Skin 70
Sleep and Fatigue 70
Snacks 71
Spicy Foods 72
Sports Nutrition 72
Stress 74
Sugar 74
Taste and Flavor 75
Vegetables 75

Vegetarian Eating 76
Vision 77
Vitamins 77
Weight Gain 78
Weight Loss 79
Women's Health 82
Yeast Infections 83

Appendix: How to Spot Nutrition Misinformation 85
References 89
Index 91

Introduction

FROM THE EARLIEST DAYS of recorded history about 10,000 years ago, people have tried to link food to health, energy, and vitality. No science existed to help our ancient ancestors. Instead they experimented. In time, they learned to identify poisonous plants from those that could nourish them—and to prepare foods they hunted.

Through circumstance, and sometimes coincidence, people found their own ways to choose, prepare, and preserve foods as nourishment. They devised ideas about what and how food could make them sick. They endowed some foods and food practices with magical and ritualistic, as well as religious and symbolic, qualities. And so, foodlore, or beliefs, practices, and traditions about food, began.

Some early recorded food beliefs suggested both health benefits for the living, as well as tranquillity and happiness for the deceased. Ancient Romans, such as Nero, ate leeks several days each month to clear their voices; other Romans ate lettuce to clear their senses; and some pressed juice from artichoke hearts as a lotion for restoring hair. At one time, Romans believed that the souls of their ancestors resided in beans, so beans were eaten at funerals. Oregano was offered to gladden the spirit of those who had passed on.

Food and herbs were ascribed with medicinal qualities. Ancient Egyptians worshiped garlic, and they gave it to laborers to endow them with strength to build pyramids. At the same time, Greeks deplored garlic and compelled criminals to eat it as a way to purify themselves from crime.

In time, flowers and fruits joined herbs and vegetables for medicinal purposes. Lily of the valley, now considered harmful, was powdered and used to treat earaches, headaches, and stroke. Tincture of rhubarb was advised for indigestion and colic; fresh snapdragon tops as a cure for jaundice.

The basis of today's nutrition science has roots in early Western medicine. More than 2,000 years ago, the ancient Greek physician Hippocrates linked disease to the physical qualities of food. Advice of moderation and variety, extolled by some Greek ancients, sounds remarkably similar to nutrition guidance given today. However, specific advice about food was far from scientific—and didn't change much until nutrition began to emerge as a true science less than 200 years ago.

During the same time period, Asian teaching added to the world's foodlore. The opposite qualities of ying (bland, lower-calorie) and yang (strong, rich, spicy) in food were believed critical to harmony within the body and sometimes important to treating disease. At about the same time, the system of "hot" and "cold" foods developed in the Middle East, Europe, and later in Latin America. The idea of "hot" and "cold" didn't refer to the temperature or spiciness of food, but instead to its perceived function in the body. For example in Mexico, rice was considered "hot" and connoted strength, while beans were considered "cold," connoting weakness. In some cultures, these food classifications continue today.

In the last century, knowledge of nutrition finally began to reveal the composition of foods. At the end of the eighteenth century, scientists were just beginning to learn about the role of food as fuel for the body. By the early nineteenth century, *A Guide to Domestic Cookery*, published for American homemakers, explained that "ripened" bread took on more oxygen, or healthy gas, increasing "nutriment" by 20 percent and giving a much greater degree of cheerfulness ... and "a much greater flow of human spirits." And the same book offered a folk remedy for an earache: "Soak the feet in warm water; roast an onion and put the heart of it into the ear as hot as can be born and bind roasted onions on the feet."

Only within the last 100 years have we begun to understand the link between food chemistry and food's health-promoting qualities. Some old food remedies are respected today, as we've finally learned their scientific explanations. For example, lemons and potatoes were recognized for preventing scurvy because they contain vitamin C, fruits and vegetables were considered healthful, and many herbs used in home remedies are part of modern medicine.

Food traditions and legends—as well as myths—reflect our culture. Many foods are invested with symbolism. Others help define our cultural celebrations. Still others have religious meanings. As long as these food traditions and lore don't contradict wise health practices, they remain a respected, often joyous, part of our lives.

Food folklore has been part of history for all time. Each era and each culture has discarded some foodlore, kept some, and introduced their own. Many of these ideas had no basis in science; some have proven neutral. And some foodlore eventually has been proven helpful, and as science has emerged, has become part of sound nutrition advice.

Even today, myths encircle our beliefs about food and its health-promoting qualities. As we look at the past, we may smile about many notions about food and health. Yet it's often hard to sort through the facts and fallacies about food that engage our attention today. Clever phrases, wishful thinking, pseudo-science, media hype, and testimonials—rather than sound science—often lure consumers to today's nutrition mythology.

To Separate Fact from Fiction

Food myths and misinformation aren't likely to disappear in the near future. As long as people want solutions to health concerns—especially quick, easy, even magical answers—food myths will appear and perhaps make headline news. Many myths will be recycled with new names, and perhaps new promises. As scientific knowledge about the functional qualities of food and herbs gets unlocked, popular advice may get ahead of the science that backs it up.

Before you accept the "latest" health or nutrition advice—and spend money on what may be ineffective remedies—make sure the advice is backed by science, not simply the next generation of foodlore. These 10 signs of "junk science" should send up a red flag of suspicion.

1. Recommendations that promise a quick fix
2. Dire warnings of danger from a single product or regimen
3. Claims that sound too good to be true
4. Simplistic conclusions drawn from a complex study
5. Recommendations based on a single study
6. Dramatic statements that are refuted by reputable scientific organizations
7. Lists of "good" and "bad" foods
8. Recommendations made to help sell a product
9. Recommendations based on studies published without peer review
10. Recommendations from studies that ignore differences among individuals or groups

Source: Food and Nutrition Science Alliance (FANSA)

Your best defense is healthy skepticism and taking time to be well informed. The next time you're lured by the promotion of a nutrition product, regimen, service, treatment, or device, put these "10 signs of junk science" into action. Do this by arming yourself with the checklist of questions in "How to Spot Nutrition Misinformation" on page 85. You'll be more likely to make an informed decision.

When You Need Sound Advice

To help you sort food facts from fiction, seek the advice of qualified experts. A registered dietitian (RD) or dietetic technician, registered (DTR) are among the professionals who are reliable sources of nutrition information and advice on eating and health. Your health, and that of your family, depend on sound guidance!

Tales
and
Truths

Aging and Longevity

Can taking a vitamin E supplement delay aging or get rid of wrinkled skin?
There's no conclusive evidence that nutrient supplements, including vitamin E, can stop or reverse the aging process. However, antioxidant vitamins, such as vitamin E, play a role in protecting you from some health problems that come with aging, such as cancer, cataracts, and heart disease. Ongoing research is exploring the possibility that vitamin E protects against Alzheimer's disease.

Will ginseng help you live longer?
Ginseng, which is a plant root, has been promoted as a life extender, aphrodisiac, and cure-all for almost everything, from memory loss to menopause to stress to chronic ailments. The reported benefits may come from a placebo effect; few human studies show true benefits. Taken over time, high intakes of ginseng may be linked to anxiety, breast pain, dangerous changes in blood pressure, sleep loss, and tranquilizing effects.

➤ *See Memory, Phytochemicals, Skin.*

· ·
Tradition and legend...
Eating a food you haven't tasted before prolongs your life by 75 days, according to an old Japanese saying.[1] What a great reason to try new foods!
· ·

Alcoholic Beverages

Does red wine protect against heart disease?

There's no conclusive answer. However, recent research suggests that a moderate amount of any alcohol, including wine, beer, and hard liquor, may help lower the risk of heart disease. ("Moderate" is no more than two drinks a day for men, and one for women.) A moderate amount possibly may help increase HDL- or "good" cholesterol, or prevent "bad" or LDL-cholesterol from forming in the body. And alcohol may boost the body's natural clot-dissolving or clot-preventing enzyme temporarily. Protecting your heart isn't a good reason to start drinking alcohol, however.

Myth: An alcoholic drink warms you up in cold weather.
Fact: Actually, the reverse is true. Alcoholic drinks tend to increase the body's heat loss, making people more susceptible to cold.

Myth: A drink or two gives you a "lift."
Fact: In truth, alcohol is a depressant, not a stimulant. The initial "lift" is often short-lived. Instead, alcohol may reduce concentration, coordination, and response time.

Myth: Beer is less intoxicating than hard liquor.
Fact: In the amount typically consumed—a 12-ounce can of beer, a mixed drink with 1 1/2 ounces of 80-proof liquor, or a 5-ounce glass of wine—the alcohol content, and probably the effect, are the same.

➤ *See Breast-Feeding, Caffeine, Colds and Flu, Dehydration, Dietary Supplements, Sleep.*

Tradition and legend...

Ancient Persians ate five almonds to prevent hangovers.[2] For Romans and Greeks, celery was thought to cure a hangover. By the late 1800s, celery still had a medicinal use, advertised by Sears, Roebuck & Co. as a celery tonic to calm the nerves.[4]

Anemia

Myth: Anemia is the reason for that "run down" feeling.
Fact: Perhaps, but you may be overworked and under-rested instead. A little more sleep and relaxation may do more to give you a

pickup than anything else. Anemia that causes fatigue usually is diagnosed by a blood test.

Myth: An iron deficiency always causes anemia.

Fact: Sometimes, but not always. Anemia isn't a disease but instead a symptom of several health problems. It occurs when red blood cells don't have enough hemoglobin to carry oxygen to cells for energy production. Iron is an essential part of hemoglobin, so an iron deficiency is one cause. There are other causes: blood loss, deficiencies in folate or vitamin B_{12}, and defects in blood cells or body processes that use iron.

Are eggs a good iron source?

Eggs do provide iron, but less than l milligram per large egg, mainly in the yolk, compared with 3 milligrams of iron in 3 ounces of broiled sirloin. However, the non-heme iron in eggs isn't absorbed as easily as heme iron in meat, chicken, or fish. To help your body use non-heme iron, team it up with other foods: vitamin C-rich fruits and vegetables, or meat, poultry, or fish. For premenopausal women, the recommendation is 15 milligrams of iron daily.

Will eating blackstrap molasses prevent anemia?

Along with other food sources of iron, blackstrap molasses can contribute non-heme iron to your diet. One tablespoon contains 3.5 milligrams of iron. But it's not in a form that's as readily used. To get the most benefit, blackstrap molasses needs to be consumed in meals with vitamin C-rich fruits and vegetables, or meat, poultry, or fish.

➤ *See Vegetables.*

....

Tradition and legend...

According to an old household remedy, anemia could be cured by sticking a long iron nail into an apple. After it sat overnight, the nail was removed and the apple was eaten.[3] It's hard to say how much iron that really provided. However, when foods high in acid, such as tomatoes, are cooked in cast iron pots, some iron does transfer (leach) into the food.

....

Appetite

Does your stomach shrink when you eat less?
No. Even though your stomach can expand to handle large amounts of food, it doesn't stretch out indefinitely. As food passes to your intestines, the stomach goes back to its normal size. When you cut back on the amount of food you eat, your stomach keeps its normal size.

➤ *See Fiber, Snacking, Weight Loss.*

Tradition and legend...
To the ancient Greeks, parsley was thought to promote appetite, and even bring good humor.[4] Perhaps that's why even today, a sprig of parsley brings appeal to a meal.

Arthritis

Myth: A copper or brass bracelet can relieve or cure arthritis by drawing pain out of the body.
Fact: The ill-thought myth credits magnetic properties of metal as the cure-all. No scientific evidence supports this view.

Myth: You can ease arthritic pain by avoiding eggplant, potatoes, and tomatoes.
Fact: None of these foods appears to promote joint pain. And no evidence shows that eliminating them prevents or relieves pain either. Smart advice: for relief, aim for a healthy weight to ease the load on weight-bearing joints.

Is glucosamine effective for treating arthritis?
As yet, research is limited on the effectiveness of glucosamine as a treatment for arthritis. Some of the reported studies have shown positive results, but the studies have only lasted a few weeks. Glucosamine products appear to be safe, but their purity, as sold in the United States, is unknown.

➤ *See Heart Health.*

Body Weight

Myth: For some people, everything eaten turns to fat!

Fact: It may seem that way for those who get frustrated over trying to lose weight. However, body fat is formed only when the total energy from food—whether it's from carbohydrate, protein, or fat—exceeds the amount used for daily living and physical activity.

Myth: Obesity is hereditary.

Fact: Genetics certainly play a role. But the causes are far more complex than genes alone, or for that matter, how much and what you eat. Weight problems often run in families, partly because eating and lifestyle habits are similar. Differences in metabolic rate, physical inactivity, and other psychological, social, and lifestyle factors all play a role.

Myth: People with weight problems are just lazy.

Fact: Overweight people may be more sedentary. But that doesn't mean they lack energy, motivation, or ability. Instead, holding back from physical activities may come from feeling self-conscious.

Myth: Overweight people eat more food than slim people.

Fact: In fact, the reverse may be true. Slim people are often more physically active, so their bodies need more food energy. And if their food choices are lower in calories, perhaps with more low-fat foods, they may eat larger amounts. For maintenance, muscle uses more calories than body fat does; that's another reason that a slimmer, muscular person may need more food energy than an overweight person with less muscle. In addition, slim people also may "run" at a faster metabolic rate, meaning they burn more energy just to keep their bodies working.

Myth: Fat kids grow up to be fat adults.

Fact: Not necessarily. It's true that childhood weight problems have reached an alarming level. Eleven percent of kids ages six to 17 are considered overweight—up from five percent a decade ago. Excess weight during childhood can have both physical and psychological consequences. But overweight kids aren't destined to be overweight adults. With plenty of physical activity and a healthful eating pattern, they often grow into their weight during the rapid growth spurt of puberty.

Tales and Truths

Myth: There's an ideal weight for your height.
Fact: Not true. Each person is an individual with a different body size and shape, and different bone structure and muscle composition. For good health, there's a weight range that's probably best for you to maintain good health. It's probably not the same weight as your favorite media personality or best friend.

Does body fat burn more energy than muscle?
Actually, the reverse is true. The more muscle you have, the more calories you need just to maintain your weight.

Myth: You're fat if you can pinch any skin or if your flesh jiggles.
Fact: Your body needs some body fat to stay healthy! The layer of fat under the skin insulates you from cold and heat and protects your vital organs from injury. Even firm flesh can jiggle a bit when muscles are relaxed.

➤ *See Child Feeding, Infant Feeding, Weight Gain, Weight Loss.*

Tradition and legend...
In former centuries, extra pounds of body weight related directly to prosperity. (Just walk through an art gallery for a view of past beauty!) Those who weighed more were considered blessed with money to buy food. Perhaps they also had a lifestyle that didn't require physical labor.

Bone Health
Myth: Taking a calcium supplement prevents osteoporosis.
Fact: Many things contribute to bone health. A calcium supplement only addresses one nutrition factor: inadequate calcium intake. Gender, body size, race, smoking, exercise levels, estrogen levels, and heredity each play a role, too. A calcium supplement can help promote bone health. But for most healthy people, eating enough calcium-rich foods can provide an adequate amount of calcium.

Myth: Women don't need to worry about calcium intake if they take estrogen.
Fact: Whether they take estrogen or not, women need adequate amounts of calcium to slow bone loss during and after menopause. Their bodies also need calcium to carry out other important functions. The recommendation for women through age 50 is 1,000

milligrams of calcium daily. After that, 1,200 milligrams of calcium are advised to help maintain bone mass. As a point of reference, an 8-ounce glass of skim or whole milk has about 300 milligrams of calcium.

> See Dairy Foods, Physical Activity.

Breast-Feeding

Myth: Women with large breasts produce more milk.
Fact: Breast size has no bearing on the success of breast-feeding or the volume of milk produced. Breast size depends on the amount of body fat and fibrous tissue, not glandular tissue which produces milk.

Will breast-feeding prevent food allergies in the baby?
Maybe so. For those with a family history of allergies, breast-fed babies are less likely to have food allergies—if breast-feeding continues for at least six months.

Myth: Breast-feeding is an effective form of contraception.
Fact: Although breast-feeding does decrease fertility, it's not 100 percent effective for contraception.

Myth: Beer or wine before breast-feeding promotes a mother's milk supply.
Fact: That's a "wives' tale." In fact, alcoholic beverages may negatively affect the let-down reflex. And some alcohol may pass into a mother's milk.

Myth: A mother needs a healthful diet to make nourishing milk for her baby.
Fact: Even poorly-nourished mothers produce nutrient-rich milk for their babies, but mothers may produce less milk, depending on how poor the diet is. The real "cost" of a poor diet comes at the expense of the mother's health. For example, if calcium intake comes up short during breast-feeding, calcium reserves in a mother's bones are used to make breast milk. A varied and well-balanced eating plan during breast-feeding days benefits the mother more than the baby.

Do mothers who drink a lot of milk have colicky babies?
Maybe—if the baby is sensitive to protein in cow's milk. When breast-feeding mothers drink cow's milk, the protein passes into

her breast milk. Some studies have found that mothers of colicky babies have higher levels of cow's milk protein in their breast milk than mothers whose babies are not colicky. To check, stop eating milk, dairy foods, or whatever food seems to cause the problem for a short time to see what happens. And talk to your pediatrician. What seems like colic from something you eat might just be a coincidence. Most babies don't react to what their mothers eat.

Caffeine

Myth: Drinking coffee helps "sober up" someone who drinks too much alcohol.
Fact: Coffee, or other caffeinated beverages, won't make you sober, just more awake! Only time can make someone sober. A healthy liver detoxifies about one drink per hour.

Myth: Cola is the only soft drink with caffeine.
Fact: Color doesn't indicate the presence of caffeine. Both clear and caramel-colored soft drinks may—or may not—have caffeine. And some citrus-flavored drinks have the most caffeine of any soft drink. Some soft drinks have information about caffeine on the label—either stating "no caffeine" or listing caffeine on the ingredient list.

Myth: Chocolate has a lot of caffeine.
Fact: Chocolate does contain caffeine, but not much. Compare chocolate milk and candy with a cup of coffee. Both an 8-ounce carton of chocolate milk and a 1-ounce milk chocolate bar each contain about 5 milligrams of caffeine, compared with 115 milligrams of caffeine in 5 ounces of regular-brew coffee.

Myth: Caffeine boosts physical performance.
Fact: Maybe—and maybe not. People react to caffeine in different ways. For some, it may stimulate the central nervous system, helping them feel more alert and attentive, and perhaps enhance energy level. For some athletes, it may exacerbate pre-event anxiety. It also has a diuretic effect, promoting water loss through urination, which may promote dehydration and the fatigue that comes with it.

➤ *See Chocolate, Fluids and Beverages.*

Tradition and legend...

Coffee beans, which originated in Africa, were used by Abyssinian soldiers. Roasted and pulverized, then mixed with grease, "coffee balls" were used as battle foods on short skirmishes. [2]

....

Calories

Myth: Margarine contains fewer calories than butter.
Fact: Ounce for ounce, the calorie and total fat content of regular stick margarine and butter are the same—about 100 calories and 12 fat grams per tablespoon. For fewer calories, try whipped butter or margarine. Both are whipped with air, so they're less calorie-dense.

Myth: Olive oil has fewer calories than either butter or regular margarine.
Fact: Because oils are concentrated and solid fats may have some other ingredients besides fat, olive oil has slightly more—14 fat grams and 120 calories per tablespoon. The main difference is the type of fat. Olive oil is mostly monounsaturated; butter and stick margarine, mostly saturated.

Myth: Toasting bread lowers the calories.
Fact: Calorie counters might wish that lowering calories was so easy. However, toasting only reduces the water in bread, and water has no calories. Toasted or not, an average slice of bread provides about 70 calories.

Myth: Eating grapefruit or vinegar burns calories.
Fact: This long-held myth is just wishful thinking. Digestion of any food uses a small amount of energy. But no food—or food component—can "burn up" the calories in food or "melt away" body fat. If you lose weight when you add grapefruit to your eating plan, it's probably because you're substituting it for another food that has more calories.

How many calories do you lick from a postage stamp?
According to the U.S. Postal Service, anywhere from two to ten calories per stamp. The amount depends on the size of the stamp—and whether you lick the adhesive well or just give it a "dab." For a large stack of holiday greeting cards, use a sponge or self-adhesive stamps instead!

Tales and Truths

There's no fat in soft drinks, so where do the calories come from?
Calories in soft drinks come from sugars, which is one form of carbohydrate. Carbohydrates and proteins provide 4 calories per
gram, while fats provide 9 calories per gram. Fat isn't the only
nutrient that provides calories!

➤ *See Cholesterol in Food, Fat, Fast Food, Food Labeling, Fruit*
and Fruit Juice, Grain Products, Healthful Eating, Snacks,
Sugar, Weight Gain.

. . . .
Tradition and legend...
Not long after potatoes were brought from the Americas to
Europe 500 years ago, they were banned for fear of causing lep-
rosy, as well as sold at high prices as a cure for impotence. By
the 1700s, the Irish were among the first to recognize their
value as an important source of nourishment.[2, 5]
. . . .

Cancer
Myth: Taking large amounts of antioxidants—beta carotene and vitamins
C and E—prevents cancer.
Fact: There are many unknowns in cancer prevention. Yet, scientific studies suggest that consuming larger amounts of antioxidant
vitamins may offer protection. Currently, there's not enough evidence to suggest how much, and large doses may have dangerous
side effects. Because protection may come from many substances
in food, not just antioxidants, following an overall healthful eating plan and lifestyle is the best advice.

Myth: Food additives cause cancer.
Fact: Food additives are highly regulated, and only those judged
to be safe are allowed in the food supply. By law, no additive
known to cause cancer in animals or humans can be put in food
in any amount. If found to be safe, the Food and Drug Administration decides what types of foods the additive may be used in,
in what amounts, and how it must be indicated on the food label.

Do vitamin B17 supplements prevent cancer?
No. In fact, vitamin B_{17}, also known as laetrile, isn't a vitamin at
all! Instead it's a substance derived from the inedible pits of apri-

cots and the stones of other fruits. Laetrile also contains cyanide, which can be lethal. Fortunately, the edible portion of fruit itself doesn't contain laetrile.

Will drinking green tea prevent cancer?

One component of green tea—an antioxidant called polyphenol—is receiving special attention for its potential anti-cancer factor. There's some evidence that tea, especially green tea, reduces the risk for some cancers, heart disease, or high blood pressure. But there's still more to be learned. There are no known negative effects of drinking green tea.

Can shark cartilage keep tumors from forming?

Shark cartilage, which is actually gristle, provides calcium. However, there are no scientific findings for supporting an anti-cancer claim. In fact, it may be harmful to pregnant women or those recovering from wounds, surgery, or heart ailments since it may affect the development of blood vessels. It may not be absorbed anyway.

Myth: Eating high-fiber cereals prevents colorectal cancer.

Fact: High-fiber cereals—especially those high in insoluble fiber from whole-wheat products, wheat and corn bran—certainly help reduce the risk of colorectal cancer, but by themselves they won't prevent it. So don't feel you're home free just because you eat a fiber-rich cereal for breakfast. From a dietary standpoint, eating plenty of fruits and vegetables and following a low-fat eating plan also are important in reducing the risk.

> ➤ *See Irradiation, Physical Activity, Phytochemicals, Women's Health.*

Carbohydrates

Is a high-carbohydrate eating plan okay for someone with insulin resistance?

There's a lot to learn about insulin resistance. But research suggests that a more moderate fat intake (30 to 35 percent of calories from fat, rather than less than 30 percent) might be beneficial for people with insulin resistance. That means that calories from carbohydrate would be somewhat less than typically recommended, too. With insulin resistance, insulin can't help glucose to pass from the blood to body cells where energy is produced or stored as glycogen for the future. A glucose tolerance test can help diagnose insulin resistance. There are no obvious physical symptoms. It's most common among those with Type 2 diabetes, and for many with problems of high blood pressure, heart disease, or obesity.

➤ See Fiber, Food Labeling, Sugar, Weight Loss.

Child Feeding

Myth: Kids need to "clean their plates."
Fact: Pressuring kids to eat everything on their plate puts too much emphasis on food—and may lead to a habit of overeating. (Perhaps portions were too big for kids' appetites anyway.) This kind of pressure can lead to power struggles between parents and kids. As children self-regulate how much food they eat, they're also learning to listen to their body's appetite signals. It's up to parents to decide which foods to provide as children learn to make choices.

Are food jags harmful?

Actually, they're more frustrating to parents than harmful to young children. Wanting the same food over and over usually lasts for just a few days—not long enough to be a real concern. Parents can offer other foods alongside that food to encourage variety. If whole categories of food are rejected for more than two weeks, it's appropriate to talk to the doctor or a registered dietitian.

Myth: Children must eat three meals a day.
Fact: For growth, health, and energy, children need a varied, balanced eating plan for the day, not necessarily for each meal. The Food Guide Pyramid, shown on page 53, shows the variety of food-group foods children need. It makes no difference if kids consume those foods in three meals or six mini-meals.

Myth: A low-fat diet is right for all kids.
Fact: Before two years of age, children need enough fat to support brain development, their rapid growth, and their active lifestyle. Between ages two and five, parents can help children cut back gradually on fat. By age five, the Dietary Guidelines for children are the same as those for adults: no more than 30 percent of total calories from fat. Children also need concentrated energy from moderate amounts of fat for their high levels of physical activity.

By choosing foods with fat from different sources, children get the two fatty acids (linoleic and linolenic acids) that are essential for their growth and health. A very-low-fat diet can be harmful.

Myth: Overweight children need to follow a weight-loss diet.

Fact: Restricting calories may be harmful to growing children. They may miss out on the nutrients they need for growth and health, as well as the food energy needed to help them learn, develop, and explore their world. Usually, healthful eating habits and plenty of active play help children grow into their healthy weight, without further weight gain. Most kids don't need to follow a special diet. If parents are unsure, they need to talk with their physician or a registered dietitian for guidance.

➤ *See Body Weight, Dairy Foods, Food Allergies and Sensitivities, Snacks.*

Chocolate

Does drinking chocolate milk make kids "hyper"?

There's no scientific evidence that the sugar or the very small amount of caffeine in chocolate milk are linked to hyperactivity.

Myth: Some people are chocoholics.

Fact: It's true that some people do have a stronger preference for chocolate than others, but true addiction is not possible. While popping chocolate candies may become a high-calorie habit, eating chocolate itself can't become truly addictive.

➤ *See Caffeine, Skin.*

. . . .

Tradition and legend...

Chocolate, which first came from the Americas, was considered a gift from the gods in pre-Columbian times—and a form of currency. In the 1500s, Native Americans served it to honor their European guests, the explorers who came to what is now Mexico.[6]

. . . .

Cholesterol in Food

Myth: Trimming fat takes all the cholesterol from meat—so does removing poultry skin.

Fact. Trimming away fat and removing poultry skin reduces, but doesn't eliminate, cholesterol or fat. Dietary cholesterol is found in the lean muscle and fat in both meat and poultry.

Myth: Seafood and chicken have "good" cholesterol; meat and cheese have "bad" cholesterol.

Fact: Cholesterol in food is neither "good" nor "bad." In food, it's all the same. So-called "good" (HDL) and "bad" (LDL) cholesterol refers to cholesterol in the body, not food.

Why doesn't cholesterol provide calories? Fat does.

Although similar in structure to fat, cholesterol isn't broken down during digestion, so it can't supply food energy, or calories.

Myth: Stick margarine has more cholesterol than soft margarine.

Fact: Neither one contains cholesterol, since they're made from vegetable oils. Only foods of animal origin have it; both butter and lard contain cholesterol. Although they're still high in fat, margarine and vegetable oil are both cholesterol-free.

> ➤ *See Alcoholic Beverages, Eggs, Food Labeling, Heart Health, Meat.*

Colds and Flu

Myth: A "nip" of brandy helps fight a cold.

Fact: To the contrary, alcohol can reduce the body's ability to fight infectious bacteria. It also may interfere with medication.

Will chicken soup make you well?

So they say, perhaps as a comfort food offered by a caring friend or family member. Hot soup, or perhaps any warm liquid, feels good inside as the warmth spreads through the body. Chicken soup itself is a nourishing and typically easy-to-digest food when you're ill, and the warmth may help open the nasal passages. Whatever the reason, enjoy it on your way to recovery.

Myth: Feed a cold, starve a fever...or starve a cold, feed a fever.

Fact: Either way, it's a myth! To fight infection, your body needs a supply of nutrients to build and maintain your natural defenses.

A day's eating plan with variety and balance are as important as ever. Extra rest and plenty of fluids helps, too.

Myth: Large doses of vitamin C cure the common cold.

Fact: An adequate amount of vitamin C is important for fighting infection. However, scientific evidence doesn't justify taking a large dose of vitamin C, perhaps from a vitamin supplement, on a regular basis to boost immunity. Extra amounts may have a mild antihistamine effect, perhaps shortening the duration of a cold and making the symptoms more mild.

Will echinacea cure a cold or flu?

Classified as a medicinal herb, echinacea may offer some physical benefits to the immune system during illness. However, effectiveness of this herbal supplement varies with the form and dosage taken. People with health problems affecting the immune system, such as HIV, need to be especially cautious.

Is lobelia safe for reducing cold and fever symptoms, or treating sore throats or other respiratory ailments?

No, it's not safe! In low doses, this medicinal herb may work as a nicotine-like stimulant, dilating lung bronchi and aiding breathing. However, the Food and Drug Administration reports that taking lobelia may have harmful side effects: breathing problems, rapid heart beat, sweating, coma, and death from larger doses.

Will taking zinc lozenges help you recover faster from a cold?

Zinc is an essential trace mineral, involved in many body processes. Recently, zinc gluconate lozenges have been promoted to shorten the duration of a cold. So far, studies on their effectiveness are limited. And large amounts of zinc can be toxic, perhaps impairing copper absorption, weakening immune response, and lowering HDL-cholesterol levels. Until more is known, consume adequate amounts of zinc from food sources, including red meat and seafood.

➤ *See Dairy Foods, Food Safety and Foodborne Illness, Taste and Flavor.*

Tradition and legend...

An old Russian "wives' tale" advises a hot, moist mixture of oat-meal and dry mustard, spread on the chest, to ward off pneu-monia.[7]

Dairy Foods

Myth: You shouldn't drink milk if you have a fever.

Fact: A person's body temperature has no bearing on drinking milk. Whether a person is healthy or sick, the nutrients in milk promote health. There is one caution however. Calcium in dairy foods and calcium supplements can block the absorption of tetra-cycline-based antibiotics. Take antibiotics 1 hour or more before or after consuming calcium-based products.

Myth: Milk is just for kids. Adults don't need it.

Fact: The nutrients in milk—calcium, phosphorus, protein, vita-mins A and D, riboflavin, others—are for everyone! Kids need plenty of calcium because their bones are growing longer and stronger. Children ages 4 to 8 are advised to consume about 800 milligrams of calcium a day; from ages 9 to 18, about 1,300 mil-ligrams of calcium. Adults need calcium to keep their bones strong and slow the natural bone loss that comes with aging. The advice for adults is: before age 50, 1,000 milligrams of calcium daily, and after that, 1,200 milligrams daily.

Myth: Cottage cheese is a great calcium source.

Fact: Cottage cheese does supply calcium, about 65 milligrams in a half-cup serving. However, it has less than other dairy foods: about 300 milligrams of calcium in 8 ounces of milk or yogurt, and about 200 milligrams of calcium in 1 ounce of cheddar cheese.

Myth: All molds on cheese are harmful.

Fact: Not usually. But just to be safe, discard one inch of the cheese on the sides where mold appears. On mold-ripened cheese, such as blue, Gorgonzola, or Roquefort cheese, mold gives the distinc-tive flavor. It's okay to eat unless the color and pattern of the mold differ from the usual blue or green veins, or if the cheese has furry spots, or white, pink, blue, green, gray, or black flecks. Then dis-card it. Toss moldy soft cheese, such as cream cheese or Brie, too.

Myth: On a low-fat diet, you need to avoid dairy foods.
Fact: For milk, yogurt, and cheese, you have plenty of choices, including reduced fat, low-fat, and fat-free dairy foods. Regardless of fat content, they're great sources of calcium, protein, and other nutrients your body needs.

Myth: Milk causes cotton mouth or mucus.
Fact: So-called "cotton mouth" describes a dry mouth with thick saliva, or a feeling of mucus. The condition has nothing to do with milk. For public speakers, emotional tension may instead play a role. With colds, milk may simply coat mucus in the mouth and throat, making it seem thicker. And for athletes, the amount of water lost during competition may be a factor.

➤ *See Chocolate, Food Allergies and Sensitivities, Minerals, Processed Foods, Sleep and Fatigue, Sports Nutrition, Women's Health.*

Dehydration
Myth: Sucking ice can help prevent dehydration.
Fact: Ice may cool you down, but a few cubes probably won't provide enough fluid to prevent dehydration.

Myth: Cold beer is a great fluid replacement on hot summer days.
Fact: Not so. Alcohol is a diuretic, which increases urine output and so promotes dehydration. It may help quench your thirst, but it's not the best fluid replacement when you're sweating already.

Myth: You don't need to worry about dehydration during cold weather.
Fact: Dehydration is an any-season issue. Even in the cold, people perspire, perhaps from shoveling snow, outdoor sports, or being bundled up to stay warm. Inside, dry, heated air evaporates moisture on skin so fluids are just as important in the winter.

➤ *See Fluids and Beverages, Sports Nutrition.*

Dental Health
Myth: Bleeding gums mean you're not getting enough vitamin C.
Fact: It's possible, but not likely, unless you have a severe deficiency. Most cases of bleeding gums come from poor oral hygiene. Brushing your teeth along the gumline and flossing regularly helps keep gums healthy and free of bleeding.

Myth: Eating sugar causes tooth decay.

Fact: Any carbohydrate—starches and sugars—can mix with bacteria to form acids that damage teeth. So eating a candy bar may not promote cavities any more than crackers. The longer any carbohydrate comes in contact with teeth, the greater the chance for decay. And whether or not you get cavities depends on many factors—and not just what you eat. Heredity, as well as the composition and flow of saliva, are factors. So is the care given to teeth and the frequency of brushing and flossing.

Myth: Sugar-coated cereals promote tooth decay.

Fact: From an oral health standpoint, there's little difference between the cavity-promoting potential of carbohydrates in cereal itself or in the sugar coating. Presweetened or not, the cavity factor depends on how long cereals stick between teeth or in the crevices of molars.

➤ *See Snacking.*

· ·

Tradition and legend...

About 150 years ago, a simple remedy believed to relieve a toothache was rubbing the cheek with a soft, moist paste of ginger.[8]

· ·

Depression

Will St. John's wort cure depression?

St. John's wort may help relieve some symptoms of mild depression, perhaps by affecting levels of serotonin, which is a chemical in the brain. Research is still being conducted on its effectiveness and potential uses. Its use also makes skin more sensitive to sunlight. It should never be taken with prescription antidepressants, or used to treat severe depression.

Diabetes

Myth: Sugar causes diabetes.

Fact: It's true that people with diabetes cannot use sugar in a normal way. However, the causes of diabetes are complex and related to genetics, body weight, illness, and just getting older. Sugar itself does not cause diabetes. But food, along with physical activity and perhaps medication, are part of the management of diabetes.

Will pectin supplements help control blood sugar levels?

Because pectin is a soluble fiber, it may help control blood glucose levels and help lower blood cholesterol. However, you don't need a supplement to do that. Oats, beans, apples, carrots, citrus fruits, and bananas all contain pectin, too. And they deliver other nutrients—and flavor—along the way!

Myth: People with diabetes can eat complex "carbs" but not sugar.

Fact: It's true that people with diabetes can't use energy nutrients, including carbohydrates, in the normal way. When the body doesn't produce enough insulin or can't use it properly, glucose accumulates in the blood, and blood sugar levels rise. Sugars, and complex carbohydrates in starchy foods, actually have a similar effect on blood sugar levels. People with diabetes need to space their meals and snacks. And they need to balance all kinds of carbohydrate-rich foods, including pasta, rice, bread, vegetables, and other starchy foods, with the proteins and fats in their eating plan.

Myth: Honey is natural and won't raise blood sugar levels.

Fact: Natural or not, honey is basically sugar, which acts like other sugars. Like sugar, 1 tablespoon of honey counts as 1 carbohydrate exchange. The term *exchange* refers to a system of grouping foods according to their calorie and nutrient content; foods on a specific exchange list can be substituted for each other. Exchange lists are used to plan diets for people with diabetes.

Can people with diabetes have as many sugar-free cookies as they want?

Sugar-free cookies certainly aren't a "free" food. Even though they have no sugar, they do contain carbohydrates so they count toward starch exchanges.

➤ *See Physical Activity.*

Tradition and legend...

Some cultures practice "sympathetic" medicine, believing that like cures like. For example, eating an animal organ improves the function of that same type of human organ. So, eating animal pancreas is believed to enhance insulin production, while

Tales and Truths

pork brain is believed to improve intelligence, and chicken feet, to strengthen feet.[9]

···

Dietary Supplements

Myth: Natural vitamins are better absorbed—and better for you—than synthetic vitamins.
Fact: In most cases, your body can't tell the difference. The chemical makeup is the same. Vitamin E and folate seem to be exceptions. Vitamin E in its natural form may be better released, while synthetic folate is better used by the body. So-called "natural" products often cost more than the synthetic product.

Myth: A vitamin supplement can make up for a poor eating plan. It has all the same "stuff."
Fact: No supplement can make up for an ongoing pattern of poor food choices. Supplements may supply some vitamins and minerals, but not all the components that food supplies. A varied and balanced eating pattern is your best bet for getting the nutrients you need for health.

Myth: A daily nutrient supplement is your best insurance for consuming enough vitamins and minerals.
Fact: Supplements don't provide the full array of nutrients, including vitamins and minerals, and other substances, such as fiber and phytochemicals, that food supplies. The best advice: follow the guidance of the Food Guide Pyramid. See Healthful Eating on page 52 for Pyramid advice.

Myth: A vitamin pill protects against the harmful effects of smoking or drinking too many alcoholic beverages.
Fact: No supplement or eating regimen protects against the harmful effects of either one. However, smoking does increase the body's need for vitamin C. And drinking excessive amounts of alcohol can interfere with the body's use of some nutrients.

Myth: If some vitamins are good for you, more is even better!
Fact: Each vitamin has specific functions in your body. The amount you need is relatively small. Following the advice of the Food Guide Pyramid usually provides enough. Megadoses, more than 100 percent of the nutrient's Daily Value, from vitamin supple-

ments probably won't do anything more for you. Besides being a waste of money, large doses may be toxic, or harmful, unless prescribed by a doctor to prevent or treat certain health problems. For example, large doses of vitamin B$_6$ may cause irreversible nerve damage; too much vitamin C may cause kidney and bladder problems.

Myth: Some supplements detoxify your body.
Fact: There's no evidence that any supplement can do that—nor should it. That's an internal job, already handled by your liver and kidneys. The liver breaks down toxic by-products of metabolism, and kidneys remove them through urine production.

> ➤ See Aging and Longevity, Bone Health, Cancer, Colds and Flu, Depression, Diabetes, Digestion and Digestive Problems, Energy, Fiber, Heart Health, Memory, Minerals, Muscles, Phytochemicals, Sex and Fertility, Sports Nutrition, Stress, Women's Health.

Digestion and Digestive Problems
Do spicy foods cause ulcers?
No. Food choices neither cause nor cure ulcers. Most ulcers are caused by bacteria called *Helicobactor pylori*, which are treated with antibiotics. Unless spicy foods—or any foods—cause repeated discomfort, there's no need to avoid them.

Myth: Enzyme supplements aid digestion.
Fact: For most people, the body makes enough enzymes to digest food. A lactase deficiency is one of the few exceptions; a lactase supplement, taken with dairy foods, aids digestion of milk. And, when eating legumes, some enzyme supplements may help reduce gas from forming. However, most enzyme supplements are broken down in your own digestive tract before they can work as digestive enzymes.

Myth: The stomach can't digest carbohydrates and proteins at the same time. You need to separate foods such as fruits from the meal.
Fact: First off, you couldn't separate one nutrient from another even if you wanted to. Most foods are mixtures of several nutrients. Regardless, your stomach and small intestine secrete different digestive enzymes to break down carbohydrates, fat, and

proteins. Those enzymes are ready and able to work at the same time!

Will fiber supplements keep you "regular"?

They may offer some benefits, but high-fiber foods should be the body's main fiber source. Many fiber pills supply only small amounts of fiber, compared to the amount in food. Those with more fiber may keep your body from absorbing important minerals. And, over time, your body might depend on them. Better advice: high-fiber food first!

Is aloe vera juice an effective laxative?

It's true that aloe vera often works as a laxative, but not always gently. It's not appropriate for regular use. With a regular, high-fiber diet and plenty of fluids, a laxative probably won't be needed anyway.

Myth: Highly-seasoned foods cause heartburn.

Fact: A food or type of food may promote heartburn by stimulating acid production in your stomach. When stomach acids back up into the esophagus, you may feel pain or discomfort. Foods with a lot of acid, such as citrus foods, as well as fatty foods and highly-seasoned foods, may also cause discomfort. You may be able to prevent heartburn caused by certain foods by taking an over-the-counter product that neutralizes the acid in these foods.

Will ginger relieve nausea, indigestion, or motion sickness?

Maybe—if taken as symptoms start to occur or before traveling. The reason? Ginger, an herbal product, may help neutralize stomach acids by promoting the secretion of saliva and digestive juices. Too much ginger may cause heartburn or aggravate other health problems.

Myth: Drinking milk causes constipation.

Fact: Not true. Constipation can have many causes. Drinking milk isn't one of them. Depending on the reason for the problem, drinking plenty of water and eating high-fiber foods, such as whole-grains, vegetables, fruits, and legumes, might ease the symptoms.

➤ See *Food Safety and Foodborne Illness, Infant Feeding, Legumes.*

Tradition and legend...

A typical Japanese breakfast includes pickled plums and hot tea to prevent constipation.[1] In the U.S., prunes, which are dried plums, are often consumed for the same reason.

Eggs

Myth: Brown eggs are better for you than white ones.

Fact: The color of the shell has no relation to an egg's nutritional value. Varying from white to deep brown, shell color depends on the breed of the hen.

Myth: Fertilized eggs are more nutritious than unfertilized eggs.

Fact: Not really. The difference in nutrient content is too small to make a difference.

Why would some eggs have more omega-3 fatty acids?

The difference comes from the feed. Flaxseed is high in omega-3 fatty acids. When flaxseed is used as feed for hens, the content of omega-3s in eggs goes up.

➤ *See Anemia, Cholesterol in Food, Fat, Heart Health.*

Tradition and legend...

In many parts of Europe, burying an egg laid on Good Friday or Easter Sunday in the vegetable garden or field is thought to keep hail away and protect beehives.[4] And in the Caribbean islands of Trinidad and Tobago, the shape of egg white, when added to warm water on Good Friday, predicts the future.[1]

Energy

Myth: Vitamin supplements can boost your energy level for heavy workouts.

Fact: Vitamins don't supply energy. Carbohydrate, fat, and protein do. If you're already getting enough servings from the Food Guide Pyramid to meet your energy needs, there's no need for supplements. The small amount of extra vitamins—for example, B vitamins—needed to help produce more energy in the body during physical activity comes from eating more food.

Myth: A candy bar gives quick energy.
Fact: Consuming a candy bar or a sugary drink won't supercharge your body. A high-carbohydrate diet for several days before a heavy physical workout is a better energy enhancer. For endurance activities of 90 minutes or more, diluted juice or a sports drink before and during physical activity may enhance your stamina.

Does bee pollen boost your energy level?
No, and it won't improve physical performance or cure impotence, either. As sold, it's a mixture of bee saliva, plant nectar, and pollen. But it contains the same nutrients found naturally in food: starch, sugars, protein, and a small amount of fat. Some people have an allergic reaction to it.

Is spirulina a high-energy food?
Although touted to be, spirulina, a blue-green algae, has no energy-producing qualities. It does supply nutrients, including vitamin B_{12}. However, the vitamin B_{12} in spirulina isn't in a form your body can use.

Will ma huang, or ephedra, give energy or promote weight loss?
That's what claims for this dietary supplement say, so it's part of many weight-loss teas and other aids. But in fact, the risk of taking it may far outweigh any benefit. Used improperly or too long, it can have harmful side effects: high blood pressure, rapid heart beat, muscle injury, nerve damage, stroke, psychosis, memory loss, and death.

Fast Food
Myth: A fast-food fish sandwich is lower in fat than a regular hamburger.
Fact: Actually, the fat content in a plain fried-fish sandwich is about the same as a three-ounce burger, about 12 fat grams per sandwich. Add tartar sauce and the fat in the fried fish sandwich soars to about 23 fat grams. Fish itself is relatively low in fat, but frying and tartar sauce boost the fat content.

Myth: If you want a low-calorie meal, order the salad bar.
Fact: The average plate from a salad bar may have more calories than a deluxe burger, fries, and a shake—with more than 1,000 calories! The exact amount depends on the choices and portions selected. In fact, salads have been reported as the main source of dietary fat for women.

Fasting

Myth: Fasting cleanses the body of toxins.
Fact: Your liver and kidneys are your body's built-in detoxification system. The liver breaks down toxic by-products, and the kidneys get rid of them. Throughout the world, fasting is more commonly done for religious reasons, not for health reasons.

Does fasting offer a jump start on weight loss?
No, not if you want to trim off body fat! When you fast, the first weight loss is water and muscle loss. Just by eating again, water weight comes back on; however, muscle may never be replaced. Fasting deprives your body of nutrients needed for health.

➤ *See Weight Loss.*

Tradition and legend...
About 150 years ago, fasting morning and night, and drinking plenty of cold sage tea all day long was suggested as a cure for night sweats.[8]

Fat

Myth: Extra virgin olive oil has fewer calories than pure olive oil.
Fact: The calories and amount of monounsaturated fatty acids are the same, no matter what the type of olive oil: about 14 fat grams per tablespoon. The difference is the acid content. Extra virgin olive oil has less acid and a fruitier flavor than pure olive oil.

Myth: "Light" oil has less fat and calories than other oils.
Fact: In this case, the term "light" refers to the color and flavor, not the fat and calorie content. Either way, oils have about 14 fat grams and 120 calories per tablespoon. On some products, "light" may refer to less fat, calories, or sodium. Read labels carefully to learn the meaning of their claims.

Myth: To keep healthy, it's wise to eliminate fat totally from your diet.
Fact: You shouldn't, and you probably can't. Fat is an essential nutrient, which provides energy, carries fat-soluble vitamins into your bloodstream, and promotes growth, among other functions. Some health experts recommend a level of fat in the diet of about 15 to 20 percent of total calories. For many people, no more than

Tales and Truths

30 percent of total calories from total fat, and no more than 10 percent from saturated fat, are more realistic goals. These guidelines are appropriate for good health. Fat is widely available in a variety of food.

Myth: Eggs are high in saturated fat.
Fact: Eggs are high in cholesterol, about 215 milligrams per yolk. But they aren't high in fat, and don't contain much saturated fat. One large egg has about 5 grams of total fat and 2 grams of saturated fat in the yolk, and none in the egg white.

Will eating trans fatty acids cause a heart attack?
To prevent a heart attack, it's wise to focus on key risk factors, not just trans fatty acids. Trans fatty acids are created when vegetable oils are partly hydrogenated; in the process, they become more saturated. Trans fatty acids are naturally present in food, too. The best overall advice: 1) eat a diet low in total fat, saturated fat, and cholesterol—from any sources, 2) stay physically active, 3) kick a smoking habit, and 4) control high blood pressure.

Myth: You need to avoid any food or recipe with more than 30 percent calories from fat.
Fact: The 30-percent guideline applies to your overall food choices for several days—not to one food or one meal. For a 2,000-calorie eating plan, that's no more than about 67 fat grams on an average day. To clear up any confusion, the guideline is no more than 30 percent—not 30 fat grams—a day.

➤ See Calories, Child Feeding, Cholesterol in Food, Dairy Foods, Eggs, Food Cravings, Food Labeling, Heart Health, Nuts and Seeds, Poultry, Skin, Vegetarian Eating, Women's Health.

Tradition and legend...
Inuits have used seal oil as a dipping sauce for meat and vegetables. It probably served as an emergency energy source when food was scarce.[3] Although the Inuit diet was very high in fat, the rate of heart disease was very low; the high ratio of omega-3 fatty acids may be an important factor.

Fertilizers and Pesticides

Myth: Food grown in depleted soil is less nutritious.
Fact: There's no scientific evidence suggesting that crops grown in soil depleted of minerals or nutrition have fewer nutrients than those grown in fertilized soil. When soil lacks minerals or nitrogen, plants don't grow properly and may not produce their potential yield. If the soil can grow crops, the food produced is nutritious. Some variation in nutrients is normal.

Myth: Foods grown with natural, or organic, fertilizers have more nutrients than foods grown with synthetic fertilizers.
Fact: Actually, the nutrient content is about the same. Plants can't tell the difference between synthetic and organic fertilizers. Both types break down in the soil to nurture plants. Other factors, not the type of fertilizer, may affect the nutrient content of food: climate, crop handling, maturity at harvest, genetic differences, and soil conditions.

➤ *See Organic Foods.*

Tradition and legend...
In Rome, 2,000 years ago, blood and bones, rather than human waste, were used for fertilizers. And farmers rotated clover and alfalfa to nourish the soil.[10] Pre-Columbian Americans fertilized their land, too, sometimes by burying fish in the field.

Fiber

Myth: Fiber supplements or powders help you lose weight.
Fact: Probably not. They may provide some bulk, reducing your appetite—but you can't trick your appetite for the long run. And these supplements won't necessarily keep you from eating high-fat, high-calorie foods. You're better off to choose high-fiber, low-fat foods: plenty of fruits, vegetables, whole grains, and beans (legumes).

➤ *See Cancer, Diabetes, Digestion and Digestive Problems, Grain Products, Heart Health.*

Fingernails
Myth: Eating gelatin makes your fingernails strong.
Fact: That's wishful thinking! Fingernails are mainly dead proteins that get their strength from sulfur in amino acids.

Do vitamin deficiencies cause cracking or peeling fingernails?
Probably not. It's likely caused by dry skin, soap, or the way you wash your hands. The best remedy: use a moisturizer, not a vitamin supplement.

Are ridges or white marks on fingernails a sign of a nutrient deficiency?
No, instead they're often caused by a slight injury to the nail.

Fish and Seafood
Myth: Fish is a brain food.
Fact: This misbelief has been around for a long time, perhaps arising from the fact that brain tissue and fish both contain phosphorus. In fact, meat, poultry, eggs, and meat provide phosphorus, too—but they aren't considered brain foods. An overall healthful eating plan is really the best brain and body food around!

Is it safe to eat raw seafood?
That depends. To be safe, you must buy high-quality, very fresh seafood with a certified shipper's tag—or catch it in waters certified for safety. At a restaurant, it must be sushi grade or high quality, too, prepared by highly-trained chefs who know how to buy and prepare raw seafood for safety and sanitation. High-risk individuals—those with HIV, impaired immune systems, chronic alcohol problems, liver and gastrointestinal disorders, kidney disease, inflammatory bowel disease, cancer, diabetes, and steroid dependency—should not eat raw or partly-cooked fish.

➤ *See Fast Food, Food Safety and Foodborne Illness, Heart Health, Sex and Fertility.*

Tradition and legend...
Clam broth often is served at Japanese wedding banquets. The two tightly-closed clamshells symbolize the union of the couple.[6]

Fluids and Beverages

Myth: You can count on thirst as a signal to drink more fluids.
Fact: Not always true! Older adults and those involved in strenuous physical activity may not feel thirsty when they need more fluids. As an everyday precaution, consume plenty of fluids—at least 8 cups of fluids daily. Drink more during hot temperatures, and when you're physically active, even when it's cold outside.

Myth: Bottled water is healthier for you than tap water.
Fact: Both bottled and tap water are monitored carefully for quality and safety. The only real nutritional differences may be fluoride and lead. Either tap or bottled water may—or may not—be fluoridated. You need to check. In places where the lead content of water is a concern, bottled water may be a good choice since it doesn't contain lead.

Myth: Clear drinks are calorie free.
Fact: Being clear doesn't mean a beverage is simply water. It may contain sugar, other sweeteners, or artificial flavors. If so, the beverage may have calories. Check the label.

Are caffeinated drinks a good fluid replacement?
No. Caffeine in coffee, tea, and some soft drinks—as well as alcohol in beer, wine, and mixed alcoholic drinks—acts as a diuretic. It causes your body to lose water through increased urination. You're better off drinking water, juice, milk, and decaffeinated drinks.

> ➤ *See Alcoholic Beverages, Caffeine, Dehydration, Sleep and Fatigue, Sports Nutrition, Vegetables.*

Tradition and legend...

The tradition of tea drinking has been popular for more than 2,000 years in China. Contaminated water may have been one of the reasons. A hot drink made with boiled water was less likely to cause digestive problems than plain water.[10]

Food Additives

> ➤ *See Cancer, Food Allergies and Sensitivities, Hyperactivity.*

Tradition and legend...

From Pre-Columbian times until today, Mexicans inadvertently added calcium to their diet, as they prepared corn for making tortillas.[11] By soaking corn in slaked limewater, corn becomes more digestible, while adding calcium. Slaked lime, a powdery substance, differs from citrus lime juice.

....

Food Allergies and Sensitivities

Myth: A lot of people are allergic to food.

Fact: Only one in 50, or 2 percent of adults suffer from true food allergies of any kind. Among those who do have food allergies, the most common reactions are to milk, eggs, peanuts, soybeans, tree nuts, fish, shellfish, and wheat. Nonfood allergies are more common than food allergies. If you think you have a food allergy, check with a doctor, rather than making a self-diagnosis.

Are milk allergies common?

No, although one in three adults think so! A milk allergy often gets mixed up with lactose intolerance. With a milk allergy, the body can't handle casein and other protein components in milk. The immune system starts working, causing a reaction, even though the person isn't sick. With lactose intolerance, the body can't easily digest the sugar, or lactose, in milk. The body doesn't produce enough lactase, the enzyme that digests lactose. That results in varying degrees of digestive discomfort.

Do kids outgrow food allergies?

Usually they do—at least for most foods. But let your doctor decide when and if you can start reintroducing foods that have caused allergic reactions. The best place to try a food with previous confirmed allergic reactions is in the doctor's office where your child can have immediate medical attention if needed. Allergies to peanuts and tree nuts are seldom outgrown.

Myth: With lactose intolerance, people can't drink milk.

Fact: Even for people with lactose intolerance, there's no need to give up dairy foods. People with difficulty digesting lactose in milk just need to know how to manage it. In fact, 80 percent of people with this problem can drink a cup of milk without discomfort. Others might try smaller, more frequent portions; drinking milk with food; or consuming yogurt or cheese for milk's nutrients instead. They also could consume milk with lactase added or take lactase pills.

Does "Chinese Restaurant Syndrome" really exist?
The jury's still out. There's still no definitive research linking the monosodium glutamate (MSG) used in Chinese food to migraine headaches, a tingling feeling, or other symptoms. For those who report these symptoms, other components in food might be the culprit.

➤ *See Breast-Feeding, Headaches, Pregnancy, Sports Nutrition.*

Food Cravings
What causes a food craving?
Whether physiological, psychological, or both, the reasons are unclear. An overly-restrictive diet just may make certain foods, especially high-fat, high-calorie foods, more irresistible. To manage a food craving, you might eat just a small portion, even if it's higher in fat. Or eat a low-fat, low-calorie version instead.

Is there such a thing as a "fat tooth"?
Some people seem to have a craving for fatty foods, rather than having a "sweet tooth." It may be culturally conditioned, or they may like the qualities that higher-fat foods impart, perhaps creaminess, smoothness, or crispiness. Some studies suggest that on-again, off-again dieting may amplify a fat craving.

➤ *See Chocolate, Pregnancy, Sugar, Weight Gain.*

Food Labeling
Myth: Foods labeled as "no added sugar" have no sugar.
Fact: The claim simply means that no sugars were added during processing and packing. All kinds of foods—fruit, fruit juice, vegetables, milk, grain products—contain sugars as a natural food component. That's why the Nutrition Facts panel shows how many grams of sugar one serving contains.

Myth: "Sugar-free" or "fat-free" foods are also "calorie-free."
Fact: Not necessarily. Calories come from other carbohydrates, fat, and protein. A "sugar-free" food may have calories from fat, and a "fat-free" food may have calories from carbohydrate. Either way, you're wise to read the Nutrition Facts panel of the food label to find the calories per serving.

Myth: A food that's labeled "98% fat-free" has just 2 percent of its total calories from fat.
Fact: Actually the percent refers to weight, not calories. However, if a food makes a "fat-free" claim, it can't have more than 3 grams of fat per serving. To be sure, read the Nutrition Facts label to see just how much fat is in a serving.

Are foods labeled as "light," or "lite," also low in fat?
Not necessarily. This claim on a label might mean that the food has one-third fewer calories or 50 percent less fat than the traditional version. A "low-calorie" or "low-fat" food with 50 percent less sodium might also be called "light."

Myth: Foods labeled "cholesterol-free" are also "fat-free."
Fact: That's not always so. Cholesterol is present only in foods of animal origin, such as meat, poultry, fish, eggs, and dairy foods. Fat comes from both animal and plant sources of food.

➤ *See Fluids and Beverages, Healthful Eating, Salt and Sodium.*

Food Preparation
Will meat tenderizers break down your stomach lining?
No! It's true that meat tenderizers work as enzymes, breaking down tough connective tissue. When cooked, the tenderizer loses its ability to tenderize meat, or break down protein, any more. Regardless, digestive juices would break down the enzymes so they couldn't damage your stomach lining.

➤ *See Grain Products, Healthful Eating, Microwave Cooking.*

- -

Tradition and legend...
During Medieval times, Anthimus, a Greek physician, believed food played a role in health...with recipes to show how to use medicinal spices in cooking.[4]

- -

Food Safety and Foodborne Illness

Myth: It's okay to thaw meat or poultry on the counter. Cooking makes it safe.

Fact: It's not okay. Even if it feels cold to your touch, bacteria can multiply as meat or poultry thaw and the temperature rises above 40°F. On a whole bird or piece of meat, bacteria multiply on the outer surfaces. In ground meat and poultry, bacteria can multiply inside and out! Cooking may not destroy all bacteria—especially if it's not thoroughly cooked. Remember to cool leftovers in the refrigerator—bacteria can multiply while a food cools too.

Myth: You can't refreeze meat.

Fact: Although the quality may suffer, it's okay to refreeze meat—with caution. If it still has ice crystals and has been kept in the refrigerator for one day or less it's safe to refreeze. Be aware that the quality may not be quite as good. Your best bet: cook it first, then refreeze it.

Will antibacterial products guarantee food safety?

Antibacterial products may slow or stop bacteria from multiplying; however, they don't destroy bacteria immediately. You still need to wash utensils, cutting boards, dish rags, and other kitchen utensils—and your hands—with hot, soapy water after they come in contact with food.

Myth: If a food tastes okay, it's safe to eat.

Fact. For safety's sake, you can't depend on a food's taste, odor, or appearance. Bacteria in food can multiply in just a few hours, giving no detectable signs of contamination. If you're not sure, toss without tasting!

Is food safe if you remove the moldy part?

No, toss it out! Even if you can't see other signs of contamination, mold is a signal that a food is no longer to safe to eat. Cheeses (except for soft cheese) are exceptions; just cut off one inch of cheese on the sides where mold appears.

Are diarrhea, chills, an upset stomach, and a mild fever always symptoms of the flu?

Often, but not always. Flu-like symptoms instead may be caused by foodborne illness from eating contaminated food. In fact, many

Tales and Truths

cases of foodborne illness go unreported because people often attribute their symptoms to the flu.

Myth: Drinking alcohol with raw oysters ensures that they're safe to eat.
Fact: No scientific evidence suggests that downing a shot of vodka after eating a raw oyster kills any bacteria. Neither does the dash of hot sauce on raw oysters. To ensure the safety of raw seafood, it needs to be certified for safety, then handled properly.

Myth: Wooden cutting boards are safer than plastic ones.
Fact: Either type needs to be kept very clean—wash in hot, soapy water or in the dishwasher—so bacteria from one food doesn't transfer to another. However, plastic cutting boards have a safety edge. Bacteria in raw meat doesn't stay on plastic as it does on wood, and plastic boards are easier to clean. If you like a wooden board, use it just for meat and wash it carefully—for your own safety.

Myth: Spices such as cloves destroy bacteria in meat or poultry.
Fact: Nothing makes up for proper cooking. Bringing meat and poultry to a safe internal temperature destroys bacteria. In fact, spices can mask off-flavors that may accompany food spoilage.

➤ *See Dairy Food, Fish and Seafood, Food Storage, Infant Feeding, Irradiation.*

....
Tradition and legend...
Until the 1300s salt was used in very large amounts as an additive for preserving meat, fish, and vegetables. It was so desirable that even in Roman times, soldiers received "salarium," or salt as money, in payment. That's where the term "salary" was derived.[4]
....

Food Storage
Myth: It's not safe to refrigerate food in the can after opening.
Fact: As long as the can is covered well with plastic wrap or foil, then refrigerated, the food remains safe for several days. There may be a slight change in quality (flavor or color), however.

➤ *See Food Safety and Foodborne Illness.*

Tradition and legend...

Hanging an ear of corn in your kitchen or bedroom is said to bring good luck and fertility.[4]

Fruit and Fruit Juice

Myth: Juice-sweetened fruit spread has fewer calories and sugar than regular jam.

Fact: Not so. They're about the same. From either source—fruit juice or refined sugar—sugar has about 13 grams of carbohydrate (sugar) and 50 calories per tablespoon. To compare, check the Nutrition Facts on the label. If you want less sugar, look for reduced-sugar products.

Will drinking fruit juice make kids fat or stunt their growth?

A recent national survey done by the U.S. Department of Agriculture shows no link between drinking 12 ounces or more of fruit juice daily and either childhood obesity or short stature. Many kids don't even consume the equivalent of 6 ounces (1 serving) of fruit juice daily. As a general guideline for health, children need 2 to 4 fruit group servings daily.

Myth: The terms "sugar" or "water" on juice labels means they have fewer nutrients.

Fact: In fact, naturally-occurring sugar and water are part of all juices. Some juices have more natural sugars than others, although naturally-occurring sugars are not listed as ingredients. Sweeteners and water may be added to tart juices, such as cranberry, to make them more enjoyable. Regardless of whether water and sugar are added, juice still retains its nutrients.

Myth: Juicing makes fruits and vegetables healthier for you.

Fact: No, although some juice-machine promoters may leave you with this perception. Juices typically offer the vitamins and minerals found in whole vegetables or fruit. But they may have less fiber because some gets left behind in the pulp. In spite of cure-all claims, changing the form of food by juicing can't deliver added benefits. But for some people, it may be a way to include fruits and vegetables in an eating plan. Regardless, juicing offers a food that provides both nutrition and great taste!

Does drinking cranberry juice protect you from a urinary tract infection?
Maybe so. Urine is normally free of bacteria. But bacteria that can travel from the rectum into the bladder may cause an infection. Drinking cranberry juice cocktail may help decrease the amount of bacteria in the urine, according to recent research. Regardless, if symptoms of a urinary tract infection last longer than 24 hours, you're wise to see a doctor. A doctor may prescribe antibiotics, drinking large amounts of water, and a heating pad. Symptoms include a frequent, urgent need to urinate, painful urination, cloudy urine, lower back or abdominal pain, and blood in the urine.

➤ *See Calories, Processed Foods, Vegetables.*

. . . .
Tradition and legend...
Two thousand years ago during China's Ch'in dynasty, eating peaches at just the right time was supposed to save the body from corruption—until the end of the world! Even today, many Chinese eat shoutao, meaning "long life peach," to celebrate birthdays. Shoutao are steamed rolls, shaped like peaches. [6]
. . . .

Grain Products
Myth: Brown bread has more fiber than white bread.
Fact: Whole-grain breads are browner and typically contain more fiber than breads made with refined white flour. However, being "brown" doesn't make bread whole-grain! It may contain mostly refined flour. The rich brown color may come from caramel coloring, which is listed on the label's ingredient list. To find a fiber-rich bread, check the label's Nutrition Facts panel and the ingredient list for breads made mostly with whole-wheat or other whole-grain flour.

Myth: Washing rice gets rid of some calories.
Fact: Washing rice before or after cooking it doesn't get rid of calories. But it does wash away some important B vitamins, added to enrich and fortify rice.

➤ *See Calories, Sports Nutrition, Weight Gain.*

Tradition and legend...

Throwing rice at newlyweds probably came from China, where rice symbolizes fertility.[1] According to Filipino custom, grains of rice are presented to a new business to help ensure the success of the venture (the business will never "go hungry").

●●

Hair

Myth: Hair analysis can diagnose a vitamin or mineral deficiency.

Fact: Except to detect poisonous elements, such as lead or arsenic, hair analysis isn't a valid way to check nutritional status. Among the reasons, hair-care products affect its composition. Age and gender also affect hair quality. And the condition of hair strands varies along their length.

●●
Traditions and legends...

According to an old "wives' tale," to cure baldness you can burn hazelnuts, mash them with suet, then smear the mixture on the head.[7]

●●●

Headaches

What foods cause headaches?

Probably none, at least not directly. No scientific evidence shows that any food is a direct cause of headaches. However, some food components—either naturally present or added—may trigger headaches. A combination of environmental, emotional, and physical factors probably cause most headaches.

Will taking feverfew relieve headaches?

That's the claim for this medicinal herb, but further study is needed. It also can cause mouth ulcers. Until more is known, there's no recommendation or safe dosage for ingesting feverfew.

➤ *See Food Allergies and Sensitivities.*

●●
Tradition and legend...

Ancient Romans thought that walnuts were a miniature version of the human brain with the outer green husk as the scalp, the hard shell as the skull, and the nut as the two hemispheres of the brain. With this similarity, they declared that walnuts could cure a headache![6]

Health Foods
Myth: Health foods are more nutritious than other foods.
Fact: Any food can be called a "health food." The nutritional quality of foods sold in health food or natural food stores isn't necessarily any better than those sold in traditional supermarkets. Both types of stores sell nutritious foods than can fit within an overall healthful eating plan.

➤ *See Organic Foods.*

Tradition and legend...
The pomegranate, a many-seeded fruit, is a very old Semitic symbol of abundance, fertility, and life. Later this fruit traveled eastward from the Middle East to Asia. There it became the custom to throw a pomegranate on the bedchamber floor of newlyweds, spilling its seeds as a blessing for many children.[2]

Healthful Eating
Myth: Some foods are "good" for you; others are "bad."
Fact: No single food is "good" or "bad" for you. In a healthful eating style, any food can fit! In fact, what you eat during the whole day or several days is what really counts. Consider this: a diet that contained only a few nutritious foods, such as broccoli or milk, wouldn't be healthful if that's all you ate. And, in moderation, snack foods, such as candy and soft drinks, can fit into a healthful eating style—if you eat enough food variety overall, without too many calories.

Myth: If you follow the Food Guide Pyramid, you eat too much food—and too many calories!
Fact: If you choose mostly lean and low-fat foods, eating minimum serving amounts from the Pyramid can add up to just about 1,600 calories. With that, you can get food variety with enough of the nutrients your body needs. Adding fats, oils, and sugars from

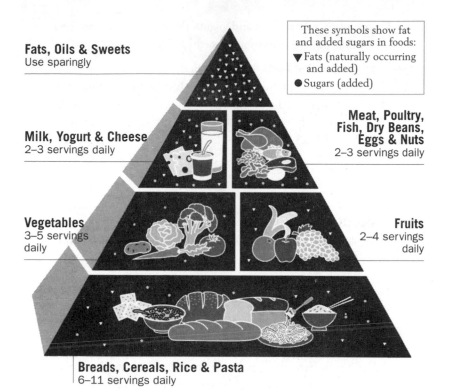

Fats, Oils & Sweets
Use sparingly

These symbols show fat and added sugars in foods:
▼ Fats (naturally occurring and added)
● Sugars (added)

Milk, Yogurt & Cheese
2–3 servings daily

Meat, Poultry, Fish, Dry Beans, Eggs & Nuts
2–3 servings daily

Vegetables
3–5 servings daily

Fruits
2–4 servings daily

Breads, Cereals, Rice & Pasta
6–11 servings daily

the Pyramid tip adds more calories. If you need more food energy, consume more calories mostly from food-group servings.

Myth: It takes too much time to eat healthy.
Fact: Today's consumers have plenty of fast and healthful ways to prepare food, for example: 1) quick cooking methods, such as stir-fry cooking and microwave cooking, 2) partly-prepared convenience foods that only require assembly at home, and 3) prepared take-out foods from supermarkets and restaurants. In each case, the options can deliver variety, flavor, and nutrition to the plate.

What does the term "healthy" on food labels mean?
In truth, any food can be part of a healthful eating plan, so the term is a misnomer. However, on food labels the term "healthy" has a regulated definition. It refers to a food that's low in fat and saturated fat, with 480 milligrams or less sodium per serving, and at least 10 percent of the Daily Value of one or more of the following: vitamin A, vitamin C, calcium, iron, protein, and fiber. In addition,

Tales and Truths

many canned or frozen fruits and vegetables and certain enriched grain products can be labeled as "healthy."

Myth: Some combinations of foods are harmful.

Fact: No scientific evidence shows that food combinations are harmful. Foods that can be eaten separately can certainly be eaten together. Be aware, however, that there are interactions between some foods and medications, which may hinder or enhance the usefulness of both.

➤ *See Health Foods, Meal Skipping, Snacking, Taste and Flavor.*

· ·

Tradition and legend...
Collard greens probably were among the African plants that came to America with slaves. Today, these nutrient-rich green vegetables have become a common part of Southern cuisine.[6]

· ·

Heart Health

Myth: Fish oil supplements protect you from heart attacks.

Fact: Fish oil supplements do have omega-3 fatty acids, which may help lower your risk for blocked blood vessels, hardened arteries, and heart attacks. But no scientific data exists about the proper dosage, or the safety and effectiveness of fish oil supplements. Regardless, they can't make up for a high-fat way of eating. It's simply better to enjoy seafood itself several times a week, and eat the low-fat way. Some fish are naturally higher in omega-3 fatty acids: for example, mackerel, salmon, sardines, and tuna.

Myth: Lecithin dissolves cholesterol in arteries.

Fact: This is just one of many claims for lecithin. Others suggest that lecithin cures or prevents arthritis, skin problems, gallstones, and nervous disorders. In truth, the body makes lecithin, which is a type of fat. Taking extra amounts doesn't appear to offer benefits.

Will eating oat bran protect you from heart disease?
No single food will prevent any health problem. However, the soluble fiber in oat bran and oatmeal (beta glucan) can have a cholesterol-lowering effect if your total fat intake is fairly low—especially if blood cholesterol levels are already high. Beta glucan binds with some cholesterol in the intestinal tract and helps remove

it from the body. Soluble fibers from psyllium (another grain) and beans (legumes) appear to have a cholesterol-lowering effect, too.

Will garlic lower blood cholesterol levels?
Maybe—but there's no conclusive evidence. Some studies suggest that consuming five or more garlic cloves daily may offer benefits. However, large amounts may irritate the stomach and cause nausea. And garlic supplements (pills and extracts) don't appear to have the same effect. Until more is known, a physically-active lifestyle and a diet low in fat, saturated fat, and cholesterol is still the best advice.

Myth: The most effective way to lower blood cholesterol levels is to stop eating eggs.
Fact: Dietary cholesterol doesn't automatically turn into blood cholesterol. So eliminating eggs won't necessarily lower blood cholesterol. The amount of total fat, especially saturated fat, has a more significant effect on blood cholesterol levels than just cholesterol in food.

➤ *See Alcoholic Beverages, Cancer, Cholesterol, Diabetes, Fat, Physical Activity, Phytochemicals.*

• •
Tradition and legend...
During the Medieval Age, a mixture of honey and thyme were thought to cure heart disease.[2]
• •

Herbs and Herbal Remedies

Myth: Herbs are used in cooking every day, so they can't hurt you when taken as supplements.
Fact: Small amounts of culinary herbs certainly add flavor and enjoyment to food. Still, although used medicinally for thousands of years, the effectiveness of most herbs as dietary supplements is being researched. The safety of many herbs is uncertain or harmful, especially in large doses or when taken over a long period. As supplements, they're more concentrated, too. And some are known to interact in harmful ways with over-the-counter or prescribed medications. Until more is known, medicinal herbs should be used with caution and with the knowledge of your doctor.

Tales and Truths

► *See Aging and Longevity, Cancer, Colds and Flu, Depression, Dietary Supplements, Digestion and Digestive Problems, Headaches, Heart Health, Memory, Sleep and Fatigue.*

Tradition and legend...

In 15th and 16th century Europe, a container, referred to as a confection box, was stocked with household medicine, much like today's medicine cabinet. Typically it held 12 sugary "pills," made of honey and saffron mixed with herbs, seeds, and spices: almonds, anise, caraway, cherry kernels, cinnamon, cloves, coriander, a spicy berry of the pepper family, fennel, ginger, nutmeg, and pepper.[2]

High Blood Pressure

Myth: A no-salt diet protects against high blood pressure.

Fact: If you're sodium sensitive, then removing the salt shaker from the table does help protect against high blood pressure, or hypertension. However, sodium is the real issue, not just salt, which is 40 percent sodium by weight. Both salt and sodium are used widely in processed foods. Check labels so you consume just moderate amounts, about 2,400 milligrams daily. To help control high blood pressure, stick to your healthy weight, stay physically active, and avoid smoking.

Myth: Eating pork and other red foods causes high blood pressure. Eating acidic foods, such as vinegar, pickled foods, and lemon juice, causes low blood pressure.

Fact: Neither is true. These notions often are confused with the concept of "high blood" and "low blood," a belief among some people in the South. The belief underlying the "high blood" myth is that excess blood goes to the head when a person eats foods that are red, such as beets, carrots, grape juice, and red meat. The notion of "low blood," linked to anemia, comes from eating acidic foods. This too is an unfounded folk belief. Both salt-cured pork and pickled foods made in a brine (salt and water) need to be limited among those with high blood pressure.

► *See Cancer, Physical Activity.*

Hyperactivity

Myth: Eating sugar causes hyperactivity.

Fact: No scientific evidence links sugar to hyperactivity or to attention deficit-hyperactive disorder (ADHD). The causes of nervous, aggressive, and impulsive behavior, and a short attention span, aren't completely understood. However, a child's overall surroundings—and how he or she deals with them—are more likely to play a role.

Do food additives cause hyperactivity?

There's no scientific evidence linking food additives to hyperactivity. The Feingold diet, which restricts foods containing salicylates (present in almonds, certain fruits, and vegetables), artificial flavors, colors, and preservatives, has claimed to manage hyperactivity. However, the evidence was based only on individual cases, and sound studies have never repeated the results. Success instead may have been based on the increased attention given to the child.

➤ *See Chocolate.*

Hypoglycemia

Does sugar trigger hypoglycemia?

Not likely, although so-called health clinics may diagnose "sugar-induced hypoglycemia" and offer costly remedies. Anxiety, headaches, and chronic fatigue from a condition called reactive hypoglycemia are rare. For those who truly have it, symptoms usually appear about two to four hours after eating a large meal. The body secretes too much insulin, causing a drop in blood sugar and perhaps symptoms of shakiness, sweating, rapid heartbeat, and trembling. These same symptoms might also come from extreme hunger, which isn't necessarily a sign of low blood sugar.

➤ *See Diabetes.*

Infant Feeding

Myth: Babies can't taste.

Fact: Indeed they can taste. In fact, babies are born with an innate preference for sweet flavors. They may perceive differences in the taste of mother's milk, perhaps when strongly-flavored foods such as onions, garlic, broccoli, or beans give milk an off-flavor—and sometimes get fussy about it! Their taste buds also detect new foods when they're introduced.

Myth: Adding cereal to a nighttime bottle helps a baby sleep through the night.
Fact: That's simply a habit—learned if a bottle is offered at bedtime or naptime. To avoid tooth decay, infants, toddlers, and young children shouldn't be put to bed with a bottle of thinned cereal, juice, formula, or milk. The liquid bathes teeth and gums, promoting decay. And it may keep a baby from consuming enough of the nutrients and calories from the full-strength formula or cereal later. If a nap- or bedtime bottle is provided, fill it with plain water instead.

Myth: The earlier you start solid foods, the faster a baby will mature.
Fact: A baby's development is set by his or her genetic time clock, not when solid foods are started. Most babies aren't ready to start solids until four to six months of age. That's when they can coordinate their tongue to push food to the back of their mouth for swallowing. Starting too soon also stresses a baby's immature digestive system, so that much of what is eaten passes through to the diaper.

Myth: Iron in infant formula causes constipation.
Fact: That's a common misperception. For babies who are not breast-fed, iron-fortified formula is recommended to help keep a baby's iron stores adequate. Full-term babies are born with only enough iron stores to last four to six months. They need an adequate supply to form the hemoglobin in red blood cells that carries oxygen to every cell of their body.

Is honey and water a good cure for colic?
This is a traditional infant feeding practice for some. However, giving honey or corn syrup before a baby's first birthday can be harmful. Both can harbor spores of a toxic bacteria called *Clostridium botulinum*. For infants, this can cause botulism, a severe foodborne illness that can be fatal.

Myth: Chubby babies often become overweight adults.
Fact: Chubbiness during infancy usually isn't linked to adult overweight. Restricting a baby's food intake may cause a failure to thrive, and may keep him or her from getting the nutrients and food energy needed for growth, development, and health.

Food Folklore

Myth: Infant juices cause obesity.
Fact: Inappropriate feeding methods, not juice itself, may promote excess weight gain. Indiscriminate use of juice includes using juice as a pacifier or continuing to give juice in a bottle instead of helping infants learn to drink from a cup. Drinking too much juice may displace other nutritious foods.

➤ *See Breast-Feeding.*

Irradiation

Is irradiated food safe?
The whole intent of irradiation is to increase food safety—by destroying disease-causing parasites and bacteria such as salmonella, as well as yeasts and molds that shorten a food's shelf life. Like medical x-rays, irradiation is a safe process. And like microwave cooking, irradiation doesn't make food radioactive. Irradiation has been used to preserve dried herbs and spices for many years.

Myth: Irradiation zaps the nutrients from food.
Fact: Not true. Like freezing, canning, drying, and pasteurization, irradiation results in minimal nutrient loss. But the amount is often too small to measure. With its increased shelf life, irradiated food keeps its quality longer.

Legumes

How can you tame the gas caused by eating beans?
Several things can help: 1) drain and rinse canned beans, 2) take small helpings of bean dishes, 3) soak dry beans overnight and use fresh water for cooking them, and 4) cook soaked, dry beans well.

Tradition and legend...
In ancient times, Babylonians believed in reincarnation—and that they would be reborn either into the animal world or as fava beans.[6]

Meal Skipping

Myth: Meal skipping is good for losing weight.

Fact: Skipped meals often lead to overeating at snacktime or the next meal. As a result, meal skippers may eat more calories overall! According to studies, breakfast eaters tend to eat less fat and calories during the day, and they have lower blood cholesterol levels, too.

Myth: Skipping breakfast is no big deal.

Fact: That depends on you. Studies show that meal skipping usually affects productivity: less concentration, more difficulty with problem solving, and perhaps fatigue by mid-morning. As an adult, you may be able to overcome the effects. But kids usually can't compensate, so breakfast skipping may have a negative impact on learning.

Meat

Myth: Red meat is off limits in a low-fat, low-cholesterol eating plan.

Fact: Many cuts of red meat are as lean as chicken. As part of a healthful eating plan, lean meat contributes many essential nutrients, including iron, zinc, vitamins B_6 and B_{12}, and protein—without too much fat or cholesterol. The goal is moderation: 5 to 7 ounces of lean meat, poultry, and fish for the day. A 3-ounce serving is the about size of a deck of cards.

Myth: Game, such as venison, contains no cholesterol.

Fact: The nutritional quality of game is similar to that of other meats. As an animal source of food, game does contain cholesterol, for example, about 110 milligrams cholesterol in 3.5 ounces of venison. Lean beef has less. The confusion may stem from the fact that some game, including venison, bison, elk, moose, and squirrel, are quite lean. The fat and cholesterol contents vary.

> ➤ *See Cholesterol in Food, Food Preparation, Food Safety and Foodborne Illness, High Blood Pressure, Sports Nutrition.*

Tradition and legend...

Pigs, which symbolized fertility, were sacrificed for mid-winter drunken celebrations. The Swedish custom of a Christmas ham stems from that tradition.[12]

· ·

Memory
Will taking lecithin help prevent memory loss?

No—so find another way to keep track of your car keys! There's no conclusive evidence that any other food substance or nutrient will help boost your memory. Because your body makes lecithin, a type of fat, it doesn't appear that lecithin supplements offer any added benefits. Unsubstantiated claims for lecithin also suggest that it will lower blood cholesterol; cure arthritis, high blood pressure, and gallbladder disease; and control weight.

Will ginkgo biloba help my memory?

Actually ginkgo is just beginning to be studied. It's been purported to slow short-term memory loss that comes with aging and to treat circulatory-related symptoms, among other things. Large amounts can cause digestive problems. People taking blood-thinning medications need to be especially cautious.

➤ See Aging and Longevity.

Microwave Cooking
Does microwave cooking destroy vitamins?

Proper cooking with any method destroys some water-soluble vitamins, such as the B-vitamins and vitamin C. With microwave cooking, however, more vitamins are retained than with most other methods. The reasons? A very short cooking time, covered cooking, and little or no cooking water.

Minerals
For calcium, can broccoli substitute for 3 servings of milk?

In theory yes, but in practice, probably not. One-half cup of broccoli has 45 milligrams of calcium, compared with 300 milligrams of calcium in 8 ounces of milk. To equal the calcium in three cups of milk, you'd need to eat 10 1/2 cups of broccoli!

Tales and Truths

Myth: Calcium in food causes kidney stones.

Fact: First, only a small percent of people ever develop kidney stones. So cutting back on calcium isn't a good approach for the general population. Among those who do develop kidney stones, trying to avoid calcium isn't the best way to prevent a recurrence. Calcium is essential for healthy bones and overall good health. Instead it's best to check with a physician for other strategies.

Myth: Colloidal minerals are better absorbed than other mineral supplements.

Fact: There's nothing uniquely better about minerals sold as colloidal minerals—and there may be serious safety concerns. Colloidal minerals, which are sold in solution, claim to be better absorbed due to their small size and negative charge. Instead, absorption depends mostly on minerals the body needs. Supplements identified as "colloidal minerals" may contain minerals that are toxic, especially in large amounts: for example, aluminum, lead, mercury, silver, and strontium. And levels of calcium, magnesium, and other needed minerals are limited. It's best to consume enough minerals from food and perhaps a conventional supplement.

> ➤ See Anemia, Arthritis, Bone Health, Colds and Flu, Dairy Foods, Dietary Supplements, Hair, Infant Feeding, Salt and Sodium, Sex and Fertility, Vegetables, Women's Health.

Muscles and Strength

Myth: Extra protein, perhaps from steak or amino acid supplements, makes muscles stronger.

Fact: Only athletic training builds muscle strength and size. Consuming more protein from food or dietary supplements won't make any difference. Amino acid supplements, such as arginine, carnitine, and ornithine, won't increase the size or strength of muscles or offer other ergogenic benefits. By definition, amino acids are the building blocks of protein. Amino acids in supplements are no different, chemically speaking, from those in food. Most athletes need from 1/2 to 3/4 gram of protein per pound of body weight a day; they can get enough from their eating pattern. More than this means extra calories, which may lead to more body fat.

Food Folklore

Will creatine build muscle mass?

Creatine is an amino acid, made in the liver from other amino acids. The body probably makes enough. Scientific investigation is studying creatine's role in building muscle mass and its effectiveness as a supplement.

➤ *See Vegetables.*

· ·
Tradition and legend...

In times past, some African tribesmen ate lion flesh, believing that it gave them strength and bravery. In contrast, eating rabbit imparted weakness and timidness.[3]

· ·

Nutrition Advice

What can a registered dietitian do for you?

As professionals, they recognize that all foods can fit into a healthful eating style. They understand that there are no good foods or bad foods, only good or bad eating styles. And they value taste and enjoyment as part of healthful eating. Registered dietitians and other nutrition experts can provide advice about healthful eating based on sound science.

Myth: Credentials on a published report guarantee sound nutrition advice.
Fact: Credentials are no guarantee. Check out the advice with a qualified expert, such as a registered dietitian (RD). Find out how the nutrition claims are supported, why the advice was published, what experts think—and if the advice really does apply to you!

Nuts and Seeds

Myth: Dry-roasted nuts have less fat than oil-roasted nuts.
Fact: There may be a difference in flavor. But the amount of fat is about the same—14 fat grams per ounce. The fat comes from the nut itself. Nuts don't absorb much fat during roasting.

➤ *See Grain Products.*

Tradition and legend...

Sweetened almonds, or Jordan almonds, enjoyed at weddings, ensure the sweetness of a marriage, according to Middle East and Greek cultures.[1]

• •

Organic foods

Myth: Organically-grown foods are more healthful and safer than foods grown in conventional ways.

Fact: No scientific evidence shows a difference. Either way, the nutrition content is basically the same, as long as foods are handled properly. Organic foods are typically grown with natural pesticides and insecticides to prevent crop damage. With conventional agriculture, pesticides are carefully regulated to ensure their safe use for the environment and human health. For those who prefer organic foods, they are nutritious choices in a healthful eating plan.

➤ *See Fertilizers and Pesticides.*

Physical Activity

Myth: Heart health is the only reason adults need physical activity.

Fact: Certainly a moderately active lifestyle promotes a healthy heart. However, physical activity is also linked with a decreased risk for certain cancers, diabetes, high blood pressure, osteoporosis, and other health problems.

Myth: You're busy. Of course, you're active!

Fact: Being "busy" isn't necessarily the same as being physically active. An active lifestyle means at least 30 minutes of physical activiity on most—if not all—days of the week. Physical activity can come from sports or recreational activities, or the everyday "active" tasks of living, including walking up steps and many household chores.

Myth: Being physically active takes a lot of work.

Fact: It doesn't need to, especially if physical activity is woven into everyday life. In fact, you don't need to get an intense workout or target a specific heart rate for health benefits. Regular, moderate activity can do the trick!

➤ *See Sports Nutrition, Weight Loss.*

Food Folklore

Phytochemicals

Are phytochemicals listed as additives on food labels?

Phytochemicals are the scientific name for naturally-occurring substances in food. "Phyto-" means plant. Because they occur naturally, you probably won't see them on the ingredient list. And it's a good thing, because plant sources of food contain hundreds of different phytochemicals.

Can phytochemical supplements prevent cancer, heart disease, or other diseases of aging?

Science is just beginning to uncover the role of phytochemicals, or plant chemicals, in health. Until more is known about them—the chemical makeup of phytochemicals, the amounts in food, and how they work—specific claims or advice can't be given. However, experts do advise consuming plenty of vegetables, fruits, legumes, and whole-grain products for the potential health benefits of their phytochemicals and the other nutrients and components in these foods.

Poultry

Myth: Free-range chickens are leaner.

Fact: Not necessarily. Genetic stock, age, and growth rate have more influence on fat levels than how they were raised. In fact, coop or barnyard chickens tend to have about the same exercise levels. Older, large chickens and those that grow quickly tend to have more fat.

To reduce fat, do you have to remove skin before you cook it?

No. It's okay to leave poultry skin on while it's being cooked. That keeps it more moist and appealing. Just remove the skin before you eat it.

➤ *See Cholesterol in Food.*

Pregnancy

Myth: Avoiding certain foods during pregnancy can prevent food allergies in the baby.

Fact: There's no evidence that this practice makes a difference, and it's not advised. In fact, mothers who severely restrict their food and calorie intake during pregnancy increase the chance of having a baby of low birthweight.

Myth: Eating cornstarch, ashes, or clay may help decrease nausea, promote a healthy baby, or ease delivery.
Fact: This is an old myth that began hundreds of years ago, perhaps with the notion to ease labor, prevent birthmarks, or smooth a baby's skin. In fact, cravings for any non-nutritive substances, a practice referred to as pica, can harm both mother and baby.

Does eating for two mean twice the food?
No, an additional 300 calories a day is enough to support the extra energy needs for pregnancy. The need for vitamins and minerals goes up a little right away. Extra nutrients should come from more food-group servings, including one extra serving from the Milk Group. Plenty of folate-rich fruits and vegetables, as well as folic acid in fortified foods and supplements, also are important to prevent certain birth defects.

Is dieting during pregnancy okay?
No!! Enough food energy and nutrients are essential for the demands of pregnancy. Weight gain is more than the developing baby. Pregnancy temporarily changes a woman's body. At the end of a full-term pregnancy, most babies are about 7 to 8 pounds. The rest of the 20 or so pounds goes to the placenta, amniotic fluid, and increases in the mother's breasts, uterus, blood volume, muscle tissue, and fluid. Extra body fat is stored, too, as an energy reserve for breast-feeding later.

Why do pregnant women crave pickles or ice cream?
Whether it's pickles and ice cream, or something else, cravings and food aversions are common during pregnancy. The reasons are unclear but may be related to hormonal changes. Regardless, they're harmless unless the woman avoids whole categories of nutrient-rich foods or if she craves non-food substances.

....

Tradition and legend...
Eggplant, eaten before delivering a baby, causes difficult labor, according to Filipino foodlore.[1]
....

Processed Foods

Myth: Fresh vegetables and fruits contain more nutrients than canned or frozen.

Fact: In fact, there's little difference, depending on their handling. Because canned or frozen fruits and vegetables typically are processed at their peak, they may have even more nutrients. For fresh fruits and vegetables, the nutritional quality depends on their care after harvest, from farm to your table. If produce is stored improperly or too long, nutrients may be lost. Whether fresh or processed, you can minimize nutrient loss by storing, preparing, and handling food properly.

Myth: Unpasteurized (raw) milk has more nutrients than pasteurized milk.

Fact: Pasteurized milk is quickly heated to a temperature high enough to kill harmful bacteria, such as *Salmonella*. Any changes in nutrient content from pasteurization are insignificant, making pasteurized milk nutritionally about the same as raw milk—and from a food safety standpoint, far superior. Regardless, certified-safe raw milk isn't widely available to consumers anyway.

➤ *See Irradiation.*

Tradition and legend...

In the late 1800s, a heated battle between John Harvey Kellogg and Charles W. Post propelled their processed breakfast cereals into prominence as American "health foods," positioned to address "digestive ills," as well as prevent or cure other health conditions.[13]

Productivity

➤ *See Energy, Meal Skipping, Sleep and Fatigue.*

Protein

➤ *See Fingernails, Muscles, Vegetarian Eating, Weight Loss.*

Tradition and legend...

Insects are quite nutritious! They supply 10 percent of the quality protein consumed around the world.[14] Grasshoppers themselves are 15 to 60 percent protein. And spiders are highest in protein, pound for pound!

Salt and Sodium

Myth: A salty taste is the best clue to high-sodium foods.
Fact: Many foods high in sodium don't taste salty. Reading the Nutrition Facts on the label, not flavor, is your best guide to a food's sodium content.

Myth: People are born with a preference for salty flavors.
Fact: Not so. A preference for salty foods is learned. And if you gradually cut back on sodium in food choices, the desire for salty flavors declines.

Myth: Most sodium in food comes from the salt shaker.
Fact: Actually about 25 percent or less of sodium comes from food preparation or salt added at the table. Most sodium comes from processed foods. It's added to help preserve, add flavor, improve the texture, bind ingredients, and control the speed of fermentation (in foods such as cheese, bread dough, and sauerkraut).

Myth: Celery is high in sodium.
Fact: One stalk of celery has about 35 milligrams of sodium, which isn't very much. The overall guideline is to keep sodium intake to 2,400 milligrams or less a day.

Are "salt-free" foods low in sodium, too?
Actually, salt is made of sodium and chloride. There are many other ingredients that contain sodium, including monosodium glutamate, soy sauce, and baking powder. If a food is labeled "salt-free," it must contain less than 5 milligrams of sodium per serving, regardless of its source.

Myth: Sea salt is healthier than table salt.
Fact: The sodium content is comparable. And it offers no known health advantages. As with other types of salt, use it judiciously.

➤ *See Food Labeling, High Blood Pressure, Sports Nutrition.*

Food Folklore

Tradition and legend...
According to folklore, spilling salt is bad luck. But tossing it over
your left shoulder right away can reverse bad luck.

Sex and Fertility

Myth: Extra zinc or vitamin E improves sexual prowess.

Fact: Throughout history, products have been marketed under this
guise. However, no nutrient supplement, including zinc or vitamin E, improves sexual performance or works as an aphrodisiac.
Overall health and fitness work best!

Myth: Royal jelly improves sexual performance in men.

Fact: Royal jelly is produced by worker bees to nourish future
queen bees. There's no evidence that royal jelly offers any physical benefits to humans. Its only effect appears to be psychological. A caution: severe allergic reactions may occur in some people.

Myth: Yohimbe, an herbal product, is an aphrodisiac.

Fact: This medicinal herb, sometimes used to treat impotence, has
been shown to be ineffective. In addition, the Food and Drug
Administration cautions about its potentially serious side effects:
nervous disorders, paralysis, fatigue, stomach problems, and death.

Myth: Oysters increase sexual potency.

Fact: As a seafood choice, oysters contribute nutrients toward a
healthful eating plan. Good health itself is important for sexual
function. However, oysters don't have any unique qualities that
increase sexual potency.

➤ *See Aging and Longevity, Breast-Feeding, Energy.*

Tradition and legend...
Over the centuries, a long list of foods and herbs have made
the list of aphrodisiacs, among them almonds, anchovies, arti-
chokes, basil, brains, caviar, cherries, chestnuts, chocolate,
crabapples, dates, eggs, figs, garlic, lentils, mangoes, octopus,
peaches, pomegranates, rosemary, saffron, tomatoes, and truffles.[15]

Skin

Myth: Eating chocolate or greasy foods causes acne.

Fact: Teens especially hold this widely-held belief. However, hormone changes, not chocolate or greasy (or fatty) foods, are the usual cause of acne.

Will skin products with vitamins get rid of wrinkles?

No—if only they could! Vitamins, amino acids, cocoa butter, herbs, or other nutrients in cosmetics and skin creams can't remove wrinkles or prevent aging skin. The one possible exception is Retin-A (derived from vitamin A), sold by prescription, which may slow the process. Although widely prescribed, there's no research on its long-term effects. And it does increase skin's sensitivity to sunlight. The best advice: protect your skin from sunlight and moisturize it daily. During pregnancy, Retin-A should only be used under a doctor's supervision.

➤ *See Aging and Longevity, Heart Health.*

· ·

Tradition and legend...

Within Native American cultures, corn has special meanings for both ritual and healing. Rubbing cornmeal on a child's skin is believed to help ease a rash. Sprinkling cornmeal around a bedside protects a sick patient from any more illness.[6]

· ·

Sleep and Fatigue

Myth: Consuming wine or another alcoholic beverage before bedtime is a sleep aid.

Fact: Although alcoholic beverages may cause drowsiness, they also interfere with normal sleep patterns. Initially, you may fall asleep more quickly, but you may not sleep as deeply or may awaken during the night.

Does melatonin protect you from jet lag?

The claim for this nutrient supplement may be partly true. However, you need far less to promote sleep than the amount sold in over-the-counter products. And there are no studies on the long-term effects, safe dosage, or interactions with food or medications. Usually the best approach is to start a trip rested, drink plenty of fluids during the flight, and try to adapt to the clock at your destination.

Will valerian root cure insomnia or relieve anxiety?
This medicinal herb may offer benefits for sleep and treating nervousness. It appears to have a mild tranquilizing effect, and may relieve muscle cramps, too. Like many other herbal supplements, recommendations for safe and effective dosage often vary by manufacturer. It should never be used when taking other sedatives or anti-depressants.

Myth: A big lunch makes you drowsy in the afternoon.
Fact: Drowsiness comes from your overall sleep habits, age, and body cycle. In fact, new research suggests that it may be normal and induced by hormones. A good antidote: get regular rest at night.

Does a glass of milk before bedtime make you sleepy?
Tryptophan, an amino acid in milk, can help make you drowsy. In theory, you'd need more milk than you could likely drink to get enough tryptophan to make you sleep. Regardless, if milk at bedtime is a comfort food that helps relax you, go for it—and reap the calcium benefits at the same time!

➤ *See Anemia, Weight Loss.*

. . . .
Tradition and legend...
Through the ages, rosemary, or "Mary's rose," was believed to keep nightmares away, ward off evil, or prevent moths. And to the ancient Romans, maids of honor carried the ever-green rosemary as a symbol of love and life.[6]
. . . .

Snacks
Myth: Snack foods are junk foods.
Fact: There's no such thing as "junk foods," just "junky" ways of eating. Any food can fit in a healthful eating plan. In fact, snacks can include any variety of foods and beverages from all five food groups.

Myth: Snacks spoil your appetite—or your kid's appetite.
Fact: Eaten two to three hours before mealtime, a small amount of food won't ruin anyone's appetite. In fact, snacks quell hunger

Tales and Truths

pains so you're less likely to overeat at the next meal. Young children often need snacks for enough food energy since they typically eat smaller portions at meals.

Myth: Snacking causes cavities.
Fact: Snacking itself won't cause cavities, but frequent nibbling can promote them. The longer and more often teeth come in contact with food, particularly carbohydrate foods, the more time bacteria in plaque have to produce acids that damage tooth enamel. Brushing after snacking and eating the whole snack at one time controls plaque attacks.

Myth: Snacking makes you fat!
Fact: The issue here is total calories eaten during the day, not how often you eat! In fact, snacking may help you control weight—if it takes the edge off hunger so you don't overeat at mealtime. For smart snacking, try to choose foods carefully to match your calorie target for the day, without going over.

➤ *See Healthful Eating.*

Spicy Foods
How can you handle the "fire" from eating hot chile peppers?
Try dairy foods! Casein, the main protein in milk, washes away the substance in hot chiles that makes your mouth and throat "burn." The seeds and inner membranes of chiles cause the most "heat."

➤ *See Digestion and Digestive Problems.*

. . . .
Tradition and legend...
In some African cultures, a husband may judge his wife's love and respect by how hot her sauces are.[12]
. . . .

Sports Nutrition
Will salt tablets prevent muscle cramps?
No, that's just a myth. Water loss, not sodium loss, causes muscle cramps, which are a symptom of dehydration. With water loss, concentrated amounts of salt cause the stomach to draw fluids from other parts of the body as they dilute the salt, perhaps causing cramping and dehydration.

Myth: Drinking milk before a workout causes stomach cramps.

Fact: Contrary to popular belief, drinking milk before physical exertion doesn't cause stomach discomfort or digestive problems. For some, discomfort could be caused by lactose intolerance instead. If so, milk can still be part of a training diet. Over time, not consuming enough calcium, a key nutrient in milk, may contribute to muscle cramps instead.

Myth: With proper training, you don't need to worry as much about fluid replacement when you work out.

Fact: Training does not protect you from dehydration! In fact, a well-trained athlete sweats more, at a lower body temperature, as a way to cool his or her body more efficiently. Everyone needs to drink plenty of fluids before, during, and after physical activity.

Myth: Except for contact sports, being leaner is better for sports.

Fact: It's true that a lean, muscular body performs better, and being lean is healthful, too. However, being too lean has consequences. Fat cushions body organs, offering protection from injury. Being too lean may cause fatigue sooner. For endurance sports, some body fat is used to supply energy. Restricting energy intake too much may create a deficiency of important nutrients, too.

Myth: After a heavy workout, you need extra vitamins.

Fact: Not true. You don't lose vitamins when you sweat! The small amount of extra vitamins needed to produce energy can come from the extra food you eat to meet your increased energy needs.

Does chromium improve physical performance?

There's no scientific evidence that taking a chromium supplement, perhaps chromium picolinate, improves physical performance ... or aids weight loss, reduces blood sugar and cholesterol, or prevents osteoporosis, as claimed. Because food choices usually supply enough, a chromium supplement doesn't appear to offer benefits. Large doses may be toxic, or harmful.

Myth: Wheat germ and wheat germ oil are good ergogenic aids.

Fact: Wheat germ does provide nutrients, including protein, B-vitamins, and vitamin E. However, it has no proven benefits for muscle building or enhancing physical performance. At the same time, there are no known side effects or adverse effects from consuming them, either.

Tales and Truths

➤ *See Caffeine, Dairy Foods, Energy, Muscles, Weight Loss.*

....

Tradition and legend...

Barley has been grown as a staple food since prehistoric times. Because it was considered to be a mild grain, athletes in ancient Greece trained on barley mush.[2]

....

Stress

Do you need "stress" vitamins when you're under emotional stress?

No. Emotional stress—from a busy, harried lifestyle—doesn't increase nutrient needs. Any claims that promote vitamin supplements for stress relief are misleading. The physical stress that comes with recovery from illness, surgery, or injury may benefit from a physician-prescribed supplement.

➤ *See Aging and Longevity, Sleep and Fatigue.*

Sugar

Myth: Honey and raw sugar are more nutritious and lower in calories than refined sugar.

Fact: Nutritionally speaking, the calorie and carbohydrate content in natural sugars and refined sugar are about the same: 4 calories per gram of carbohydrate. They're just different forms of sugar, a simple carbohydrate. Because honey is more concentrated than sugar, you can use a little less for the same sweetness.

Can you be addicted to sugar?

No. A so-called "sweet tooth" isn't a sugar addiction. Addiction is either an emotional or physical dependence or both, which can result in symptoms of withdrawal. That doesn't happen by eating sugar or any other form of carbohydrate.

➤ *See Dental Health, Diabetes, Energy, Food Labeling, Fruit and Fruit Juice, Hyperactivity, Hypoglycemia, Weight Gain, Yeast Infections.*

Tradition and legend...
According to past accounts of Hawaiian food folklore, chewing sugar cane made teeth strong and clean.

Taste and Flavor

Why doesn't food seem to have much flavor when you have a cold?
Flavor is actually a combination of several senses: smell, taste, and touch (mouth feel and temperature). A cold affects the ability to perceive all the sensations. Try this: hold your nose, and eat an onion. It may seem more like an apple than an onion. By holding your nose, you limit the smell receptors, which help perceive flavor, high up in your nasal passage.

Myth: You have to give up taste to eat healthy.
Fact: Taste and nutrition go hand in hand. Just prepare foods well to maximize their flavor. Be adventurous and try the flavors in a variety of food. Learn how to enjoy all foods—even higher-fat or higher-calorie foods in small amounts. Experiment with lower-fat versions of your favorites.

➤ *See Infant Feeding, Spicy Foods.*

Tradition and legend...
As good manners in the second century B.C., people having an audience with the Chinese emperor perfumed their breath with a clove kept in the mouth.[6]

Vegetables

Myth: Eating spinach makes you strong.
Fact: It's true that spinach does contain iron. However, oxalic acid, another food component in spinach, binds with iron, limiting its absorption. So spinach isn't the greatest iron source. Regardless, physical exercise, not iron or any other nutrient, builds muscle strength.

Myth: Beets help your body build iron-rich blood.
Fact: This myth may have its origin in the red color of beets, not their nutrient content. Beets have very little iron, which is essential to healthy blood.

Can you eat the wax on vegetables and fruit?
Yes, you don't need to peel waxed produce. Just wash it with water, brushing it to remove any dirt. The thin wax coating on cucumbers, apples, and other produce is applied after picking to help retain moisture, prevent spoilage, and protect food from bruising.

➤ *See Fruit and Fruit Juice, Processed Foods, Sodium, Weight Gain, Weight Loss.*

Tradition and legend...
Tomatoes were considered poisonous when first brought from the Americas to Europe 500 years ago. For a long while they thought the "red berries" were more appropriate for deterring ants and mosquitoes than for eating.[6]

Vegetarian Eating
Myth: Vegetarian eating is always low in fat and calories.
Fact: Often so, but not necessarily. Like any way of eating, a vegetarian eating style can include high-fat foods, including fried foods, candies, vegetable oils, and salad dressings, and for lactovegetarians, cheese. And vegetarian eating also can come up short on vitamins and minerals if there's insufficient food variety.

Myth: It's hard for vegetarians to get enough protein.
Fact: In truth, adequate protein isn't an issue for most vegetarians. Almost every food of plant origin, except for fruit, contains protein, at least a small amount. Legumes, nuts, and seeds are especially good sources. For some vegetarians, eggs and dairy foods are sources of protein, too.

Are soy products good protein sources for vegetarians?
As a source of protein, most soy products—tofu, soy milk, whole soybeans, tempeh, and products made with textured soy protein—are good alternatives to meat, poultry, and fish. For vegetarians

and non-vegetarians alike, they may have other benefits, too. People with lactose intolerance or milk allergies can choose calcium-fortified tofu and soy milk as an alternative to dairy foods. Phytoestrogens in soy products also may decrease symptoms of menopause, and reduce the risk for breast cancer, heart disease, and osteoporosis.

Myth: Plant proteins need to be carefully combined at each meal.

Fact: For complete protein, with all essential amino acids, you don't need to combine specific foods at each meal, as was once thought. Just eat different types of food during the day. Whatever amino acid one food lacks can come from other foods during the day.

Is a macrobiotic diet healthful?

Actually, it defies two principles of healthful eating: food variety and balance. A macrobiotic diet gradually eliminates food categories and restricts fluids. Eventually, only certain grains and small amounts of fluids are consumed. Not only is this approach to eating short on essential nutrients, but it also can lead to dehydration and may be life threatening.

Vision

Will eating carrots help you see better?

Yes, but not by giving you 20–20 vision. Instead, the vitamin A in carrots will help your eyes adjust to darkness and will help protect you from night blindness.

Vitamins

➤ *See Aging and Longevity, Cancer, Colds and Flu, Dental Health, Dietary Supplements, Energy, Hair, Microwave Cooking, Vision, Women's Health.*

● ●

Tradition and legend...

Oranges and lemons were put aboard sailing vessels from the mid-1700s on to prevent scurvy, a vitamin C deficiency. Vinegar, hard apple cider, and sea water were tried, too, but had no effect—because they contain little or no vitamin C.[3]

● ●

Weight Gain

Myth: A late dinner is more likely to cause weight gain than eating the same meal earlier in the day.

Fact: The clock doesn't really make a difference. It's not *when* you eat, but *what* that counts. No matter when they're eaten, calories seem to have the same effect in the body. Evidence does suggest, however, that regular mealtimes, including breakfast, reduce fat intake and minimize impulsive snacking, which results in fewer total calories.

Myth: Potatoes and bread are fattening.

Fact: That's a long-held myth. In fact, no food is truly fattening, and neither one of these by itself is high in calories. A medium potato has just 88 calories, and an average slice of bread, just 70 calories. It's the high-fat toppings or spreads that make calories add up. In one tablespoon, sour cream has 30 calories; butter or margarine, 100 calories; and regular mayonnaise, 100 calories. In the bigger picture, starchy foods, or those with complex carbohydrates, tend to be lower in calories than fatty foods.

Myth: Sugar makes you fat.

Fact: Eating too many calories from any source—carbohydrate, protein, fat, and alcohol—causes the body to produce extra pounds of body fat. Just because you like or eat sweets doesn't mean that eating sugary foods leads to overindulgence. And eating sweets won't stimulate the appetite for more.

Myth: Excess carbohydrates, not fats, cause weight gain.

Fact: If calorie intake exceeds calorie output, you gain weight—whether the calories come from carbohydrate, protein, or fat!

Myth: Complex carbohydrates make cellulite form on your thighs!

Fact: There's really no such "condition" as cellulite. Cellulite is just the term used to describe dimpled fat that may look lumpy. What you see is a fat layer with connective, fibrous-looking tissue that holds fat in place. Too many calories from any source, not just carbohydrates, may be stored on thighs and hips—or anywhere else. The precise spots depend on your own inherited tendency.

Myth: Starch blockers keep you from weight gain.

Fact: Starch blockers claim to impede the digestion of starch, a complex carbohydrate, so the sugars they're made of can't be absorbed or used for energy. The claim is unproven. And they may cause side effects such as nausea, vomiting, and diarrhea.

Myth: You'll gain weight if you give in to food cravings.

Fact: You may feel guilty, but you won't necessarily gain weight or mess up your weight-control plan. In fact, for many people a few bites of irresistible food may be okay—as long as you don't overdo. A rigid plan that eliminates your favorite foods may trigger negative feelings about sticking with a plan for healthful eating. On the other hand, if you can't stop at a handful of chips or a single piece of candy, keep them out of sight.

➤ *See Body Weight, Snacking.*

. . . .

Tradition and legend...

In Cyprus, observances leading up to Easter are filled with food traditions. After days of celebration and overeating, during the 50-day Lenten period the tables are filled with fruits, vegetables, grain products, pulses, and fish, preparing the body and mind for the holiest days of the year.

. . . .

Weight Loss

Myth: Sugar substitutes help you lose weight.

Fact: In theory, yes...if sugar substitutes help you lower your overall calorie intake, keeping it under your energy output. However, many people don't lose weight, even when they consume foods and beverages with sugar substitutes because they often replace calories saved with other foods.

Myth: You can sweat off body weight.

Fact: You can't, at least not for long! Sitting in a sauna or wearing a rubber belt or nylon clothes when you're physically active makes you perspire, so you can lose weight. However, pounds that disappear come from water loss, not body fat. In fact, every pound of weight loss after exercise-induced sweating equals two cups of fluid. As soon as you drink or eat something, pounds go right back on. Caution: trying to "sweat" weight away can lead to dehydration.

Is fasting an okay way to "make weight" for sports?

No, it's never recommended as a smart way to trim weight for sports. Fasting often causes fatigue and reduced energy stores in the body. It may cause muscle loss, dehydration, and decreased physical performance. If extreme, fasting can be fatal. For teens, there's another downside. Fasting keeps kids from getting the nutrients their bodies need for development and growth.

Myth: The right exercises help you "spot reduce."

Fact: Your body can't get rid of fat in just the problem places. As you tip the calorie balance in favor of weight loss, your body draws energy from all of its fat stores, including the problem spots. In time, fat will disappear in the "right" places.

Myth: Fat burners help you lose weight and burn fat.

Fact: Dream on! The only way to get rid of extra body fat is to use more energy than you consume. Simply put: more exercise and less calories from food.

Myth: Eating a celery stick helps you lose weight because you burn more calories than it contains.

Fact: A celery sick has about five calories. Burning that many would take about 15 minutes. Its weight loss benefit may be as a substitute for higher calorie foods.

Myth: You can lose weight while you sleep.

Fact: Sounds great! Some weight loss regimens actually offer this promise. However, your metabolic rate speeds up while you're physically active, not when you sleep. The only weight loss benefit to sleep itself is that you're not eating—unless you sleep walk to the fridge!

Myth: A high-protein, low-carbohydrate diet is a safe, effective way to burn body fat and lose weight.

Fact: Most high-protein are actually low-calorie diets in disguise. You may lose weight but not for the reasons claimed. Instead, very low calorie intake may cause weight loss, along with loss of energy. And high-protein diets may be higher in fat than you'd think. What's more, a very high protein diet puts a strain on the kidneys, as protein, rather than carbohydrate, is broken down for energy. On a low-carbohydrate diet, any rapid weight loss may be water loss, which goes right back on when a regular diet is resumed.

Myth: A high-carbohydrate diet makes you fat by raising insulin and blood sugar levels.

Fact: Too many calories, not insulin, are the reason people gain weight. A high-carbohydrate diet only makes you fat if you eat more total calories than your body burns. Insulin is simply the hormone that helps move blood glucose into cells where it's used for energy or changed to glycogen, a form of carbohydrate stored for later use.

Is a high-fiber, low-calorie diet an effective way to lose weight?

That depends. An eating plan with plenty of whole-grain foods, legumes, vegetables, and fruits can promote weight loss if it's low in calories, too. For adequate nourishment, it also needs to supply enough protein foods. An excessively high-fiber diet can cause constipation and dehydration if extra fluids aren't consumed. The best approach for weight loss and overall health is adding fiber to a healthful weight plan—one that doesn't drop below about 1,200 to 1,600 calories a day.

Can you lose weight safely by eating only low-calorie, liquid meal replacements?

A liquid meal replacement may be an occasional meal or snack. However, your body needs a variety of food-group foods for their full range of nutrients and food components—and for the enjoyment that helps you stick to your eating plan. Unlike past formulas, today's low-calorie liquid formulas have more vitamins, minerals, and high-quality protein. Regardless, the prolonged use of a low-calorie liquid diet without medical supervision can lead to fatigue, constipation, nausea, diarrhea, or hair loss.

Myth: Diet pills, which suppress appetite, are a sure-fire approach to weight loss.

Fact: Not so. Diet pills work by curbing the appetite. However, they usually work for just a few weeks until the body gets used to them. By themselves, they don't help people learn healthful eating habits for the long term. Some have harmful side effects, such as potential damage to the heart and nervous system. And they may be addictive.

Can you lose weight if you just eat rice, cabbage soup, or fruit?

Possibly, for the short-term. However, fad diets like these are hard to follow for long. They're boring. And they don't provide the full

Tales and Truths

range of nutrients the body needs for energy and health.

➤ *See Body Weight, Child Feeding, Energy, Fasting, Fat, Fiber, Meal Skipping.*

Tradition and legend...

According to Lithuanian custom, placing bread on the table upside-down is considered insulting and profane.

Women's Health

Myth: Vitamin supplements—for example, vitamin B₆ and vitamin E— relieve premenstrual syndrome (PMS).

Fact: There may be a psychological effect. However, there's no scientific evidence that taking nutrient supplements makes a difference in relieving PMS.

Myth: A daily tablespoon of olive oil protects against breast cancer.

Fact: No research indicates that any amount of olive oil added to a high-fat diet offers special protection from breast cancer. However, substituting olive or canola oil (monounsaturated fats) for butter or stick margarine (saturated fats), and cutting back on total fat to no more than 30 percent of calories from fat, may have significant health benefits.

Myth: Taking magnesium supplements wards off hot flashes.

Fact: There's no scientific evidence that magnesium, vitamin E, or other dietary supplements ward off the discomforts of menopause. Adequate magnesium does help promote bone health after menopause by helping the body use calcium properly.

➤ *See Aging and Longevity.*

Tradition and legend...

In Navajo culture, cornmeal is sacred and used in many important rituals. For the female puberty ceremony, a special cornmeal cake is prepared.[16]

Yeast Infections

Myth: Eating sugary foods contributes to fungal or yeast infections.

Fact: Candidiasis hypersensitivity, the so-called syndrome, claims that refined sugars, as well as processed foods, fruit, and milk contribute to candida. Candida is a fungus found naturally in the mouth, intestinal tract, and vagina. "Treatment" includes avoiding these foods and taking certain dietary supplements and antifungal drugs. However, according to the American Academy of Allergy and Immunology, the basis for this syndrome is speculative and unproved.

Does eating a cup of yogurt each day prevent vaginal yeast infections? There's no conclusive evidence that active cultures in yogurt offer protection from vaginal yeast infections. But the same cup of yogurt delivers 300 to 450 milligrams of calcium—great for bone health!

➤ *See Women's Health.*

How to Spot Nutrition Misinformation

Play "10 questions" when you're evaluating nutrition claims. You might spot misinformation with just one "yes" answer. Read the facts that follow to find out why.

Does the promotion of a nutrition product, regimen, service, treatment, or device...

Yes No

☐ ☐ 1. Try to lure you with scare tactics, emotional appeals, or perhaps with a "money-back guarantee" rather than proven results?

☐ ☐ 2. Promise to "revitalize," "detoxify," or "balance your body with nature"? Or does it claim to increase your strength, stamina, or energy level?

☐ ☐ 3. Offer "proof" based on personal anecdotes or testimonials, rather than sound science?

☐ ☐ 4. Advise supplements for everyone? Or recommend very large doses of nutrients? "Very large" means significantly more than 100 percent of the Recommended Dietary Allowances (RDAs).

☐ ☐ 5. Claim it can "treat," "cure," or "prevent" diverse health problems...from arthritis to cancer to sexual impotence?

☐ ☐ 6. Make unrealistic claims, such as "reversing the aging process" or "curing disease" or "quick, easy approach"?

Adapted from *The American Dietetic Association's Complete Food and Nutrition Guide* © 1996, 1998. Chronimed Publishing.

❒ ❒ 7. Blame the food supply as the source of health problems? Belittle government regulation? Or question the advice of recognized medical authorities?

❒ ❒ 8. Claim that its "natural" benefits surpass those of "synthetic" products?

❒ ❒ 9. Mention a "secret formula"? Or fail to list ingredients on its product label or to state any possible side effects?

❒ ❒ 10. Come from a so-called "nutrition expert" without accepted credentials? Does that person also sell the product?

Now Score Yourself

1. Fact. Playing on emotion or even fear is common among non-scientific pseudo-experts. Emotional words used to promote a product can be an instant tip-off to misinformation: "guaranteed," "breakthrough," and "miraculous" are used for emotional appeal.

2. Fact. Pseudo-medical jargon, such as "detoxify," "rejuvenate," or "balance your body chemistry," suggests misinformation. These terms have no meaning in physiology. To sort valid medical terms from hype, ask a credible expert to decipher any confusing terms or phrases. A supplement can't increase your strength, stamina, or energy level, either.

3. Fact. Be skeptical of case histories and testimonials from satisfied users—if that's the only proof that a product works. Instead look for medical evidence from a reputable institution or qualified health expert. Without scientific evidence, a reported "cure" may have other causes. Sometimes the ailment disappears on its own. The "cure" actually may have a placebo effect; its benefit may be psychological, not physical. The person may have been misdiagnosed in the first place. And even chronic ailments don't always have symptoms all the time.

4. Fact. For the record: Everyone doesn't need a vitamin supplement! A varied, balanced eating plan with enough servings from the Food Guide Pyramid provides the nutrients most healthy people need.

For most people, there's no added benefit to taking more than

100 percent of the RDAs for vitamins and minerals. To the contrary, taking too much of some nutrients may be harmful.

5. Fact. No nutrition regimen, device, or product can treat all that ails you. And they can't cure many health conditions, including arthritis, cancer, and sexual impotence. Even when they're part of credible treatment or prevention strategies, nutrition factors are typically just one part of overall health care.

6. Fact. Claims that sound too good to be true probably are. But that's what people want to hear. Misinformation thrives because people want simple cures and magic ways to change what's imperfect.

7. Fact. Providers of misinformation often belittle the regular food supply, government regulation, and the established medical community. Instead they call for "freedom of choice"…and describe unproved methods as alternatives to current proven methods. Be aware that some alternatives may be unsafe, ineffective, or untested. Among proven methods, you'll find choices.

8. Fact. There's nothing magical about products promoted as "natural." From the standpoint of science, the chemical structure of natural and synthetic dietary supplements is essentially the same. And the body uses them in the same manner. Herbal products aren't necessarily safe just because they're "natural." Some substances found in nature can have potent, drug-like effects.

9. Fact. By law, a medication must carry product information on its packaging. That includes the product's ingredients, use, dosage, warnings and precautions, and what to do if adverse reactions occur. However, misleading products or regimens seldom report all this information, including potential side effects or dangers.

10. Fact. Be wary when someone tries to diagnose your health status, then offers to sell you a remedy—especially if a costly regimen of products from a single manufacturer is "prescribed." Be wary of the methods used to assess your health, too. Many invalid tests may be hard to distinguish from the legitimate clinical assessments. Those to be suspicious of include hair analysis, iridology, and herbal crystallization analysis, among others. Get an opinion from a qualified health professional before getting these assessments or making changes based on the results.

References

General References

Duyff, Roberta Larson. *The American Dietetic Association's Complete Food & Nutrition Guide*. Minneapolis: Chronimed Publishing, 1996, 1998.

Ethnic and Regional Food Practices — A Series. Chicago: The American Dietetic Association, 1989–1998.

American Dietetic Association. *Vitamins, Minerals and Dietary Supplements*. Minneapolis: Chronimed Publishing, 1999.

References for "Tradition and legend..."

1 Kittler, Pamela G. and Sucher, Kathryn. *Food and Culture in America: A Nutrition Handbook*, 2nd edition. Belmont, CA: Wadsworth Publishing Company, 1998.

2 Lehner, Ernst and Lehner, Johanna. *Folklore & Odysseys of Food and Medicinal Plants*. New York: Tudor Publishing Company, 1962.

3 Deutsch, Ronald M. and Morrill, Judi S. *Realities of Nutrition*. Palo Alto: Bull Publishing Company, 1993.

4 Toussaint-Samat, Maguelonne. *A History of Food*. Cambridge, MA: Blackwell Publishers, 1994.

5 Tannahill, Reay. *Food in History*. New York: Crown Trade Paperbacks, 1988.

6 Root, Waverley. *Food*. New York: Simon & Schuster, Inc., 1986.

7 Chalmers, Irena. *The Great Food Almanac*. San Francisco: Collins Publishers, 1994.

8 Child, Lydia Maria. *The American Frugal Housewife*. Boston: Carter, Hendee, and Co., 1833.

9 Ma, Kee Maggie. *Ethnic and Regional Food Practices: Chinese American*. Chicago: The American Dietetic Association and the American Diabetes Association, Inc., 1990.

10 Trager, James. *The Food Chronology*. New York: Henry Holt and Company, 1995.

11 Viola, Herman J. and Margolis, Carolyn. *Seeds of Change*. Washington, D.C.: Smithsonian Institution Press, 1991.

12 Barer-Stein, Thelma. *You Eat What You Are*. Toronto: Culture Concepts Inc., 1991.

13 Deutsch, Ronald M. *The New Nuts Among the Berries*. Palo Alto, CA: Bull Publishing Company, 1977.

14 Four Winds Food Specialists, http://www.fwfs.com, 1998.

15 Wedeck, Harry E. and Evans, M. *A Dictionary of Aphrodisiacs*. New York: M. Evans and Company, Inc., 1992.

16 Pelican, Suzanne and Bachman-Carter, Karen. *Navajo Food Practices, Customs, and Holidays*. Chicago: The American Dietetic Association and the American Diabetes Association, Inc., 1990.

Index

A

acne, 70
aging, 15
alcohol, 16, 21, 22, 28, 31, 48, 70
aloe vera juice, 36
Alzheimer's disease, 15
anemia, 16–17, 17
antibacterial products, 47
antioxidants, 24
anxiety, 71
aphrodisiac, 69
appetite, 18
arthritis, 18
attention deficit-hyperactive disorder, 57

B

beans, 59
bee pollen, 38
beets, 76
beta glucan, 54–55
beverages, 43
birth control, 21
blood sugar level, 81
body fat, 20
body weight, 19–20
bone health, 20–21
bran, 54–55

bread, 50, 78
breakfast, 60
breast-feeding, 21–22
broccoli, 61
butter. *See* fats

C

caffeine, 22, 43
calcium, 20–21, 61–62
calories, 23–24
cancer, 24–25, 82
candidiasis hypersensitivity, 83
candy bar, 38
carbohydrates, 25–26, 33, 78
carrots, 77
cavities, 32, 72
celery, 80
cellulite, 78
cheese, 30
chicken soup, 28
child feeding, 26–27. *See also* infant feeding
children
  overweight, 19, 27, 49
Chinese Restaurant Syndrome, 45
chocolate, 22, 27, 70
cholesterol, 28, 54, 55, 60

chromium, 73
colds, 28–29
colic, 21–22, 58
colloidal minerals, 62
constipation, 36
contraception, 21
cotton mouth, 31
cranberry juice, 50
creatine, 63

D
dairy foods, 30, 31
dehydration, 31
dental health, 31–32, 72
depression, 32
detoxification, 35, 39
diabetes, 32–33
dietary supplements, 34–35
dietitian, 63
diet pills, 81
digestion/digestive problems,
35–36

E
echinacea, 29
eggplant, 18
eggs, 17, 37, 40, 55
energy, 37–38
enzyme supplements, 35
ephedra, 38
estrogen, 20–21
exercise, 80

F
fast food, 38
fasting, 39, 80
fat burners, 80
fat-free foods, 46
fatigue, 70–71
fats, 39–40, 63, 65, 76, 82
   calories in, 23
   cholesterol in, 28
Feingold diet, 57

fertility, 69
fertilizers, 41
fever, 30
feverfew, 51
fiber, 25, 36, 41, 50, 81
fingernails, 42
fish, 42
fish oil supplements, 54
flavor, 75
flu, 28–29
fluids, 43, 73
food additives, 24, 57
food allergies/sensitivities, 21,
   44–45, 65–66
foodborne illness, 47–48
food cravings, 45, 79
food folklore, 11–13
Food Guide Pyramid, 52–53
food jags, 26
food labels, 45–46, 53–54
food safety, 47–48
food storage, 48
free-range chickens, 65
fruit, 49–50, 67
fruit juices, 49–50, 59
fungal infections, 83

G
garlic, 55
ginger, 36
ginkgo biloba, 61
ginseng, 15
glucosamine, 18
grain products, 50
green tea, 25

H
hair analysis, 51
headaches, 51
health foods, 52
healthful eating, 52–54
heartburn, 36

heart health, 16, 40, 54–55, 64
herbs, 55
high blood pressure, 56
honey, 33, 58, 74
hot flashes, 82
hyperactivity, 57
hypoglycemia, 57

I
infant feeding, 57–58. *See also*
  child feeding
insomnia, 71
insulin, 81
insulin resistance, 25–26
iron, 17, 58, 76
iron deficiency, 17
irradiation, 59

J
junk science, 14

K
kidney stones, 62

L
lactose intolerance, 44, 73
laetrile, 24–25
laxative, 36
lecithin, 54, 61
legumes, 59
liquid meal replacements, 81
lobelia, 29
longevity, 15
low-fat foods, 60, 76
  for children, 26–27
  dairy foods and, 31

M
macrobiotic diet, 77
magnesium, 82
ma huang, 38
margarine. *See* fats

meal skipping, 60
meat, 47, 60
meat tenderizers, 46
melatonin, 70–71
memory, 61
microwave cooking, 61
milk, 30, 36, 44, 67, 71, 73
minerals, 61–62
monosodium glutamate, 45
muscles, 62–63, 72

N
nausea, 36
nutrition advice, 63
nutrition misinformation, 85–87
nuts/seeds, 63

O
oil. *See* fats
omega-3 fatty acids, 37, 54
organic foods, 64
osteoporosis, 20
overweight, 72. *See also* weight;
  weight loss
  children, 27
  infants and, 58–59
oysters, 48, 69

P
pectin, 33
pesticides, 41
physical activity, 19, 64
phytochemicals, 65
pica, 66
polyphenol, 25
potatoes, 18, 78
poultry, 47, 65
pregnancy, 65–66
premenstrual syndrome, 82
processed foods, 67
protein, 62, 76–77

R

refreezing, 47
registered dietitian, 63
Retin-A, 70
rice, 50
royal jelly, 69

S

salads, 38
salmonella, 59
salt, 56, 68
salt tablets, 72
seafood, 42
sex, 69
shark cartilage, 25
skin, 70
sleep, 58, 70–71, 80
smoking, 34
snacks, 71–72
sodium, 68
spices, 48
spicy foods, 35, 36, 72
spinach, 75
spirulina, 38
sports nutrition, 72–73
St. John's wort, 32
starch blockers, 78–79
stomach cramps, 73
stomach size, 18
strength, 62
stress, 74
sugar, 32–33, 45, 57, 74, 78
sugar-free foods, 33, 46
sweat, 79

T

taste, 75
thawing meat/poultry, 47
tomatoes, 18
tooth decay, 32
trans fatty acids, 40
tryptophan, 71

U

ulcers, 35
urinary tract infection, 50

V

valerian root, 71
vegetables, 67, 75–76
vegetarian eating, 76–77
vision, 77
vitamin B$_6$, 82
vitamin B$_{17}$, 24–25
vitamin C, 29
vitamin E, 15, 69, 82
vitamin supplements, 37, 82

W

water, 43
weight gain, 78–79. *See also*
    overweight
weight loss, 19–20, 38, 39, 41,
    60, 79–82
wheat germ, 73
wrinkles, 15

Y

yeast infections, 83
yogurt, 83
yohimbe, 69

Z

zinc, 29, 69